P9-DWF-381

SUSIE BRIGHT'S SEXWISE

Susie Bright's
Sexwise

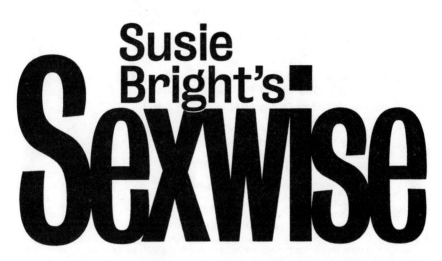

America's favorite X-rated intellectual
does Dan Quayle, Catharine MacKinnon,
Stephen King, Camille Paglia, Nicholson
Baker, Madonna, the Black Panthers
and the GOP...

CLEIS
PRESS

Copyright © 1995 by Susie Bright

All rights reserved. Except for brief passages quoted in newspaper, magazine, radio or television reviews, no part of this book may be reproduced in any form or by any means, electronic or mechanical, including photocopying or recording, or by information storage or retrieval system, without permission in writing from the Publisher.

Published in the United States by Cleis Press Inc., P.O. Box 8933, Pittsburgh, Pennsylvania 15221, and P.O. Box 14684, San Francisco, California 94114.

Book design and production: Pete Ivey
Cover photos: Jill Posener
Cleis logo art: Juana Alicia
Printed in the United States of America
First Edition.
10 9 8 7 6 5 4 3 2 1

Library of Congress Cataloging-in-Publication Data:

Bright, Susie, 1958–
    [Sexwise]
    Susie Bright's sexwise: America's favorite X-rated intellectual does Dan Quayle, Catherine MacKinnon, Stephen King, Camille Paglia, Nicholson Baker, Madonna, the Black Panthers and the GOP... / by Susie Bright. –– 1st ed.
        p. cm.
    ISBN 1-57344-002-7 (pbk.) : $10.95. –– ISBN 1-57344-003-5 (cloth) $24.95
    1. Sexuality in popular culture––United States. 2. Sex.
    I. Title.
HQ18.U5B755 1995
306.7--dc20   94-47330
                                                                                                      CIP

"Femmchismo" was originally published as the introduction to *Herotica 2,* Down There Press and New American Library, 1991, reprinted with the permission of Down There Press.

"Tie Me Up, Bog Me Down" (October 1992), "Sex and the Single Reader" (March 1992), and "The Prime of Miss Kitty MacKinnon" (October 1993) were originally published in the *East Bay Express.*

"A Pornographic Girl: Madonna's *Sex*" (Winter 1992), "Camille Anonymous" (January/February 1993), "A Taste of Power: Tasting and Talking with Elaine Brown" (March/April 1993, originally "Big Cat in the Concrete Jungle: Interview with Elaine Brown"), "Lullaby for Angela: Interview with Angela Bowie" (March/April 1993), "Better the Devil You Know: Interview with Erica Jong" (May/June 1993), "The Family Jewels: Harriet Lerner on Women, Beauty, and Anatomy" (originally "Interview with Harriet Lerner," August/October 1993) and "Fermata-cize Me!" (May 1994), were originally published in Susie Bright's "Cliterati" column in the *San Francisco Review of Books.*

"White Sex" (May 18, 1993) was originally published in *The Village Voice.*

"She Knows What She Likes: Dr. Ruth's Illustrated History of Eroticism in Classical Art" (June 1993) was originally published in the *New York Times Book Review.*

"How to Make Love to a Woman: Hands-on Advice from a Woman Who Does" (February 1994) was originally published in *Esquire.*

"Having Been Experienced: Jimi Hendrix, and Why the Little Dykes Understand" (July 1994) was originally published in *Future Sex.*

"Puberty 2001" (December 1993) and "The Pussy Shot: Interview with Andrew Blake" (September 1994) were originally published in *Playboy.*

"Adult Children of Family Values" (August 20, 1992, originally "In GOP Eyes, We All Are the Children") was originally published in the *San Francisco Examiner.*

"Dan Quayle's Dick" (Autumn 1992) was originally published in the *Realist.*

"Mommy Has to Go Out Now" (originally "Honey, I Brought the Kid," February/March 1993) and "Gaydar" (October/November 1993) were originally published in *Out!* magazine.

To Sally Binford,
Always

Contents

ACKNOWLEDGMENTS

I'd like to thank the following friends, editors, and family for all their help with this book: Lisa Palac, Bill Tonelli, Jim Petersen, Paul Krassner, Michael Goff, David Talbot, Mimi Freed, Joan Baur, The MacAdams family, Sandy Berman, Cleis Press, my agents and managers, Jo-Lynne Worley, Joani Shoemaker, Bill Bright, Jon Bailiff, Honey Lee Cottrell, Don Paul, Sarah Pettit, Jennifer Di Gioia, Shar Rednour, Christian Mann, Lupe, Rich Jensen, Michael Covino, Michael Letwin, Down There Press, David Ulin, Edward Ball, and Rebecca Hall.

9

Introduction

I GOT MY first job in the sex business during the height of the Reagan years. Instead of "Just Say No," I said, "Why Not?" I had already been a failure as a dishwasher, a well-meaning but incompetent book clerk, a less-than-charming hostess at McDonald's, and a commu- nistic ne'er-do-well at a credit service bureau. The Good Vibrations boutique in San Francisco offered me the chance to sell vibrators and dispense erotic advice in an eccentric feminist atmosphere. It was a godsend.

Our operation employed three people at the time, and catered almost entirely to a liberal, female clientele. As far as our customers were concerned—women who'd never had an orgasm, who wanted more than one, or who'd heard about our famous "try out" room— we three sexperts appeared to have achieved the pinnacle of sexual sophistication. Our reputation went beyond even that: having presumably done it all, we'd punctured or proven every sexual theory.

It is true we were well educated. If you laid out our sexual histories, we represented more sexual experience, and more variety, than your average twentieth-century woman.

But then there was our dirty little secret. There was this one year—it seemed like forever—when none of us was having sex. Of course, we didn't let go of our masturbation repertoire. We were the first to cheer for uninhibited solo sex, but still, it seemed a little weird: sex experts who couldn't get laid.

I finally bragged in ironic self-pity to a prostitute friend of mine about the Curse of Good Vibrations, and she laughed at me.

"It's not just you," she said. "I've gone for ages having sex only for money and not for pleasure. And you should see my clients: child psychologists with horrible children, divorce lawyers who can't stay married, cops whose whole families are criminals; the list goes on."

To take her explanation at face value, it seemed that the more you understood something, the less you could succeed at or enjoy it. But this conclusion didn't sit well with me. Alone in bed or not, I still felt sexually healthier, mentally more keen and clear-sighted, directly because of my sexual knowledge. It's not like I jeered at hapless passers-by, "You're sexually repressed and I'm NOT," but I felt a little cocky about it.

As it turned out, my philosophical dilemma was nipped in the bud when nature took its course. One sweaty affair and a few orgies later, I'd pretty much forgotten my quandary. The same thing happened to my coworkers. The horrible year was over; it was just an odd coincidence.

Fourteen years later, as I put together this book of essays, the quality of my sex life has come up again. The question was put to me in a recent interview by a young reporter: "Has your personal sex life improved over the decade of sexual revolution that you've been so influential in?"

It's a remarkable question. I look at the essays collected in this book, written over the past two years, and it's incredible to see how *fast* things have moved, how fast I've moved. Fame raised its pointed little head over my career, and it's hard to believe that this is the result of teaching fist-fucking workshops or demanding that pornographers be given their due. After years of gay and feminist artists talking among themselves, the mainstream has finally opened up to us like a parting sea. Figures who were considered hip and iconoclastic a month ago have suddenly become our next jeans and soda stars. My own work, which for better or worse comprised some of the more readable material of the radical fringe, is now on the celebrity gangplank. This summer I was asked at the Seattle Film Festival to model for a Starbucks Coffee company newsletter, and my only question was whether I could pose nude in the beans.

The reporter who put such a personal question to me presumed that the sexual revolution was a *fait accompli.* That had never occurred to me, especially when taking my own sex life into consideration. Yes, buying my own vibrator and having orgasms when and where I want them is liberating, but it's not my idea of uncompromised sexual freedom. My dreams of erotic liberation have been motivated by a strange mix of idealism and despair, not by consumerism and notches on my belt. I feel thoroughly repressed by my culture's notions of normality, and frankly, I'd rather die sodomizing on my waterbed than live on my knees.

It's not that I even expect to experience a sustained bohemian paradise in my lifetime. I'd just like a taste every now and then—and I have. My most memorable sexual episodes have tended to be first-time experiences: my first time with a man, my first time with a woman, my first time with a Jacuzzi jet…my first butch, my first anal sex, first group experience, first condom, first spanking…the first time I erotically tortured a lover until she begged me to let her come, the first erotic phone call I ever made to a total stranger, my first pregnancy, and, for that matter, my daughter's birth—the ultimate sexual experience. Most of these occasions happened before I was twenty. Certainly I had more sex partners when I was seventeen than any time since, so if sex is based on quantity, then I have gone downhill with each successive year.

Along those lines, if great sex is based on how many sexual positions you can assume, or how effectively you can transform your bed into a porn set, then my own sex life is mediocre. I've done lots of kinky tricks once, but I was too lazy or indifferent to repeat most of them.

What actually has improved in my sex life is how I see myself erotically—my ease with my body and my fantasies. When I was younger, I was hard on myself, judging both my desirability and the scenarios in my mind that made me hot. I thought that being "good in bed" meant being good for someone else's eyes, that perfectly staged presentations for my lovers would please them more than my own authentic excitement would. My shame about my fantasies was typical of all good little Irish Catholic girls, which was—and still is, unfortunately—awful in its influence on my adult life.

My erotic transformation was not manufactured simply. I was certainly influenced by the women's movement, which took my feminine body/beauty ambitions to task, and even more strongly by lesbian feminism, which took men's opinions off my priority list. My imagination was captivated especially by gay liberation, which teased apart my apprehensions about sexual desire.

But there are other profound reasons why I changed that have nothing to do with social movements. Number One is that I got older and realized that puberty was not the ideal erotic vantage point.

Number Two, I recognized my best lovers as my erotic mentors. I often wish I could track down the people I've lost touch with over the years to thank them for the virtual classroom that took place in our bed. My feelings were often so overwhelming, and even painful at the time, that I could never express my gratitude to my teachers except in my sexual hunger for them. In some cases, the nonsexual side of our relationship was slight, or a shambles, but that wasn't the point. Sexual illumination is as precious as any human connection.

A couple of my erotic mentors preached what they practiced, and I admired them for that. But more often, it was just Me and the Other, fucking our brains out, oblivious to the world. There was an insight to those moments that defied political argument, the truth that had no guide save my unconscious.

Finally, motherhood—from conception through pregnancy, childbirth, and my daughter's early childhood—affected my body and my sexuality like nothing else. I know that having and raising kids is the end of some women's pleasurable sex lives, but I think that demise springs more from women's social circumstances than from any physiological source. Feeling my sexuality connect with creation was thrilling, controlling that occasion was righteous, and as I say in my guide to dating mommies, if you can keep us awake, we're the love goddesses.

So, has my sex life genuinely improved because of the radical changes in sexual consciousness? Yeah, it has, and if I ever complain of dry spells or boredom, it won't be for a personal lack of sexual independence or self-esteem.

Furthermore, my life as a writer, artist, and woman has been transformed because of the very real gender and sexual revolution that started in the 1960s and has built momentum with each decade. Every time sexual speech has emerged from persecution and hiding, every time sexuality has been considered in public policy and dignified debate, my life has improved in spades. For sexual discussion to move so quickly from the criminal and pathological to the realm of the creative and political is phenomenal, a triumph of honesty and democracy over hypocrisy and elitism.

The sexual revolution is not about purchase or performance ratings. I don't give a hoot whether anybody buys a dildo, picks up a porn 'zine, watches (or makes) a dirty movie, has an abortion or in-vitro fertilization, writes an erotic short story, switches gender roles or genital expectations.

That's only a sampler of the sexual decisions and desires which, in the past, have led to punishment, disgrace and untimely death. As the late playwright Bob Chesley put it, "Prudery kills." Sexuality-as-you-like-it has been an option only to those with enough money and status to enjoy at their wealthy discretion—but not for Jane, John and Jackie Doe.

Nowadays, erotic democracy is breaking out, as the end product of the sex wars. Class distinctions and allowances for sexual freedom are still intact, but they've taken a well-deserved beating.

In part, it's just the economy doing all the talking again. Our world has no rational need for many of its anachronistic sex laws and orders; in fact, society can't afford to keep women down on the farm or all the perverts locked up. We're as productive and ambitious as anyone else, and more than a little inspired.

I wonder how dedicated the oldest ruling class (and their heirs) will be to enforcing sexual silence. History, unfortunately, has not been a series of triumphs for ever-growing enlightenment. Sexual bigotry is still very much a religion, and the extent to which zealots and defenders of the faith will fight for their prejudices is always mind-boggling.

Right now, fundamentalists of all persuasions have only been titillated with a glimpse of the largely middle-class erotic renaissance. Yes, I know they're appalled, but they ain't seen nothin' yet. Frankly, I'm sure my sex life could be better—so much better than I could possibly imagine—if their hands had never been around my throat.

Susie Bright
January 1995

I. Sex and the Single Mom

IF I WEREN'T a writer, I would have been a high school teacher. My mom was a high school English teacher, and I remember visiting her classroom once as a child and thinking how marvelous it was. The students would sing in front of her, "Mrs. Bright Is Always Right" and even if they were being sarcastic, there was real admiration in their rhyme.

I imagine I would be a good high school teacher because (a) I think school sucks, (b) I think most adults don't know what they're talking about, and (c) I think music and sex and staying up all night talking on the phone to your best friends are the greatest things on earth.

Many of my personal essays survey subjects I'd like to teach in a classroom. Cruising, for example, is something that everyone is called upon to do or to respond to in real life, and yet there is no school for neophytes except the one with extremely hard knocks. There's got to be a gentling, rather than a breaking-in for such behavior. In that vein, I offer "How to Make Love to a Woman" and "Gaydar," both of which are written from a lesbian point of view, but can be used by anyone.

Then there's motherhood. I've heard about sex education classes where each student has to stuff a pillow under his or her shirt, or carry around an egg for six weeks without breaking it. But that's foreplay. To teach a real class about parenting would be the ultimate curriculum on love, the true mystical meaning of sacrifice and gratification. It would be the mother of all boot camps.

The hardest thing about being a parent is relaxing when you feel like getting uptight, taking a time-out every once in a while, like you're always advising your children to do. That is why I wrote "Mommy Has to Go Out Now" and "Puberty 2001."

The most amazing thing about motherhood is the automatic

bullshit-detector you develop. Not only can you tell when your children are making up ridiculous stories, you can also tell when elected politicians and fearless leaders of all kinds are, in fact, lying sons-of-bitches. I never understood how there could be an organization like MADD, those mad moms against drunk drivers, while there isn't an even bigger group of pistol packin' mommas ready to burn down the halls of Congress for not doing something about child care, education, and public health. I almost had to pack a pistol and do the job myself when I was assigned to cover the last Republican National Convention, which inspired "Adult Children of Family Values."

I remember my own mother's anger about the kind of education I received. I didn't understand her fury; after all, it was "just" school, which I understood to be a glorified baby-sitting agency. Now when I contemplate putting my own daughter into those cracker-box schools with their robotic rules and discriminations, I think, "How could I do that to her?" Is it too soon for her to drop out of kindergarten and find another path? My parenting manual is obviously still in progress.

How to Make Love to a Woman:
Hands-on Advice from a Woman Who Does

As LONG AS I've been searching for promises in the backs of popular magazines, I've been drawn to that captivating title: *How to Pick Up Girls*. I'm sure you recall the ad. In addition to the untoppable come-on, it showed an average-looking bachelor carnally engulfed by a blonde, a brunette, and a redhead. His little smirk was calculated to lead us all to speculate on what his magnificent secret might be.

When I became old enough to pick up girls on my own—without a single guidebook to assist me—I thought about that cheesy Don Juan and whether I had acquired for free the wisdom his book promised for $19.95. Sometimes, during particularly blatant nights on the town, I would catch men staring at me and my latest girlfriend, their looks, a combination of envy, bewilderment, and titillation. Their eyes seemed to beg for an answer to the question, "*How?*"

Lesbians and straight men *do* have a lot in common. Both are hung up on girls. We vie for the same joy. It's only natural for each of us to wonder if the other is having more success at it. Lesbians are certainly outmaneuvered by straight men—in numbers, influence, and earning power. And of course, *you* have penises. But I often think that if I had one, I'd *really* know what to do with it. (And I don't mean cut it off.) Lesbians know female sexuality from both sides, and so we have an internal, almost incestuous intimacy with the subject. It gives us a wisdom that can't be measured.

But it can be shared.

Suppose, for example, that I wrote a book called, *How to Pick Up Girls Using the Real-Live Dyke Method*, including informative chapters on the following subjects:

The Look: For most humans, attraction begins with seeing. Look at her. All Over. Linger anywhere you like. When she notices (and she will if you're really looking), hold her eyes with yours—hold them close. Every second will feel like a minute. This is the essence of cruising, and it is the experience that virtual reality and phone sex will never replace. It is also the one moment of truth: you'll know then and there whether she wants you or not.

If she does want you, she'll be thrilled by your look, because it says to her that she has your full attention.

If she doesn't want you, she'll complain to her friends about how you "objectified" and "degraded" her, but ignore all that crap. Calling a man a sexist interloper is just a trendy way of stating an old-fashioned sentiment: "He's not my type." When a dyke gets an unwanted ogling from another dyke, we don't use political pejoratives. We just say, "Over my dead body."

Don't confuse *looking* with *watching*. "Girl-*watchers*" check out every passing femme; to *look*, as Webster so gracefully defines it, is "to exercise the power of vision."

The Touch: Lesbians, too, have probing, yearning, insistent sex organs. We call them hands. And if you have not had the pleasure of taking a woman in your hands—your thumb parting her mouth, your fingers tracing her ears, your hand curled up inside her—you are missing some of the finer points of ecstasy. Use your hands like they're your tenderest parts. The sweetest confession I ever made to a man was this: "You use your hands like a dyke."

Lesbians often say that making love to a woman feels right because "it's like touching yourself." It's a flimsy reason for choosing a partner, but a good general motto for any lover. Touch your lover the way you would touch yourself. It's about empathy, not road maps. Every part of her corresponds to a part of you.

The Surrender: Consensual rough stuff aside, the thought that emotionally mature women (meaning no nut cases) enjoy mean and nasty treatment is way outta line. Women are invariably turned on by men who can be tender—it's like watching a statue cry, very moving. She hopes she will see more of this, and so she perseveres. Most times she learns that he's only vulnerable three days out of the year, and it's not worth the other three hundred sixty-two to wait for the High Holy Days.

Personality-wise, you either have that candor and softness to express, or you don't, but sexually, anyone can lie back once in a while. Not every girl wants to get in the saddle and grab the reins, but if you have the *slightest* inkling that your woman would like to run this fuck, say a silent prayer and let her do whatever she wants.

My book would offer all that and more. But remember this bit of final wisdom: picking up girls is the easiest part of love. When it comes to seduction, you can try a dozen successful "techniques."

It's holding on to affection and lust that remains unteachable. The beginning of love is only the promise of all that's to come—for boys and for girls. Remember, it all begins with a Look, which is nothing more than a Hope—and if I can seduce a straight girl with the strength of my curious green eyes, then you shouldn't have any problem at all.

Mommy Has to Go Out Now

CALLING ALL QUEER moms! Was the last movie you happened to see a Disney cartoon? Was your last meal out Chicken McNuggets—en route to your Disney adventure?

Don't hang your head. When you can't ignore the fact that you turned to your coworkers at the end of the day and burst out, "Mommy says bye-bye!"—baby, it's time for adult entertainment.

You need to get out of the house and into somebody's pants. You need fine wines. You need meals with subtle complexity beyond the four basic food groups. You need intellectually rigorous conversation in which you are referred to by your proper first name. You need a really good fuck and maybe even a nice spanking.

From "Family Circle" to Dr. Spock, a mother can get plenty of advice about taking time for herself, particularly romantic time with either her spouse or a date. But moms need only two kernels of wisdom. The first is that your private life is precious and will make you a better mom in the long run.

The other kernel—and this is a mantra—is, "You can never have too many baby-sitters." This is particularly crucial for gay moms, because we, more often than not, rely on extended families of "aunts," "godmothers," and friends who are often the very people with whom we'd like to spend an evening out.

A mom might look around her neighborhood for a sweet sixteen-year-old who can do her homework and get a child into pajamas at the same time. But the quintessential neighborhood teenage baby-sitter may be squeamish about sex, not to mention homosexuality. Who knows what sort of parents *she* has, and how much she confides in them? The grim side of a single mom's social life is that underneath her swinging-single exterior, she is always worried that someone will try to take away her kid. The law is not on our side. No matter what contracts we've signed with donors, friendly fathers, or sperm banks, the whole area of child custody and gay parenting is up for grabs.

I take the "out-of-the-closet or out-of-my-house" approach. I told my first teenage baby-sitter that I was queer, that I wrote about sex for a living, and that my house was full of erotic art. I said, "If your parents would disapprove of your working here, or if it's not your cup of tea, then this job is not for you."

If she had hesitated even slightly, I would have gently shown her out. But like most fifteen-year-olds, she blew me out of the water. "Oh, I've seen all that before," she said, waving at my porn collection. "My mom's boyfriend gets one every time we go to Mr. Video."

I noticed the key ring she was twisting in her hand had a plastic condom pendant on it. "Some of my best friends are gay," she said, and for once, I thought that was the nicest thing I'd ever heard.

Once the baby-sitting problem is solved, the dating game becomes a lesson in the art of how to communicate with Non-Moms. Will your mystery date get into the sexy-mommy groove? Or will she be a colossal, ill-informed drag?

Of course, you could be selective and only go out with other moms. But if your kids are under five, that's physically impossible. One of you has to have a free schedule and a glimmer of spontaneity.

Let me now speak directly to those of you who are interested in dating moms. First of all, you have exceptional taste. Yes, we are more mature, we have a superb sense of irony, and if you can keep us awake, we're much hotter in bed. We are the love goddesses.

So how do you please Mommy Venus?

Take note of the following tips, designed to bring you up to speed on single-mother gestalt:

1. Do *not* ask her how she got pregnant. Lesbian Non-Moms are more obsessed with "Where's Daddy?" than anyone else outside of the Christian Right. Knock it off. If your lover's children are over age three, she's probably completely spaced on how they came into being. Don't be surprised if your mom-date says, "My daughter is from Planet X," or "I think the stork left him on the Barcalounger." Daddies come and go, but the kid is here to stay. One day Mom will tell you the whole story and it will be a testament to her trust in you.

2. Bring *Mom* a present, not the kid. Children are always getting toys from their grandparents and then spurning them for a piece of string. You don't need to suck up to your lover's children by bringing lavender teddy bears or sing-along-with-Ronnie-Gilbert albums. But ingratiating yourself to Mom is a fabulous idea. Bring flowers,

food, a good book, perhaps some semi-precious jewelry. You're driving, too, by the way.

3. Until you get to know your lover's kids, don't criticize. There is nothing more infuriating to the lesbian mom than listening to political rhetoric about how to raise her kids. ACT UP doesn't have a clue about the Terrible Twos.

This summer my daughter went to the Folsom Street Fair—a gay leather aficionados' street party—with her godmother, Honey Lee, and Honey's date. They dressed up my two-year-old in little black-leather chaps and a vest. Of course, she was adorable; a million fags were happily snapping pictures. It was one of those gay Kodak moments.

Like toddlers, one minute Aretha was a crowd-pleaser, and then some infinitesimal gesture struck her the wrong way, and it was tantrum time. There was nothing anyone could do to change her mind until she passed through the first wave of hot tears.

But wait! Here comes a lesbian Non-Mom, approaching the scene, eyeing the baby screaming her lungs out and the dyke mother-figure crouched two feet away, her mouth set in grim endurance.

"You are *abusing* this child," Ms. Well-Intentioned Idiot pronounces.

Godmom snorts, "You've been reading the wrong books."

The politically correct Non-Mom smells a good fight. She lets loose with a lecture right out of some twelve-stepper's revenge.

But wait! Aretha has stopped bawling! "Honey Lee," she cries, tugging on Godmommy's pants. "Look! See poop! Doggy poop!"

Yes, indeed, a giant black poodle with a spiked leather collar is taking a dump in front of the piercing booth, and not a moment too soon. Maybe the Non-Mom will slip in it.

Now what, you may ask, was Godmother's date doing all this time? She was soothing Honey, giving attention and sympathy to the adult at the scene of the tantrum, who is the one who really needs support.

Yes, Aretha's godmother had a real dream date, the kind of woman I'm looking for myself: a professional day-care worker. A cute dyke who works in the helping professions—you can't go wrong. Or maybe a millionairess with three teenage daughters who think babies are the best kind of fun on a Friday night! No, wait a minute, how about a six-foot Amazon who picks me up at the door, takes me into her arms, and doesn't set me down until it's time to tuck me in?

Ahhh, yes.

Nighty-night, Mommy. Sweet dreams.

Gaydar, or It Takes One to Know One

I DIDN'T ALWAYS have a lot of use for gay radar, the highly touted
psychic ability that one homosexual uses to identify another. In the
big city where I came out, if I wanted to spot someone of the gay
persuasion, I simply aimed at the nearest girl with a "Commie Dyke
Slut" button pinned to her sleeve.

"What planet did that take place on?" some of my suburban
friends have asked, and I tell them it was nothing more spectacular
than West Los Angeles in the 1970s. My initiation into lesbianism
took place in high school when a friend asked me to pass around a
petition to get Jeanne Cordova (then editor of *The Lesbian Tide)* to
speak on campus. And that was only after we imported Jane Fonda
directly from Hanoi to speak on our Girls' Athletic Field.

It wasn't until I traveled to the Midwest in 1977 that I discovered
queer bars with peepholes at the entrances and code words to gain
entry. I discovered the world of married lesbians—typified by a
woman with a husband, two point five kids, and a serious lesbo
affair going on behind the Flintstones facade. I lived in towns where
the entire lesbian social scene was a private circuit of house parties.
At my first job in Louisville, Kentucky, I was the only waitress out of a
staff of twenty-five who wasn't living with her father or her husband.
I didn't realize that my circumstances were like a lavender flag to my
coworkers—I thought I was just a role model for independent women.
But now, when I see an independent woman, I am just as whipped
up as those girls from Kentucky who didn't want to share a locker
room with me.

Sure, some people will seek out the obvious: lack of feminine
clothing, like the spinster schoolteacher who wears men's suits from
JC Penney. Or how about her favorite jukebox oldie: "I Never Loved a
Man (The Way I Love You)"?

It's easy to tell who the baby dykes are, with their homemade haircuts, or the political babes with their work shirts and steel-toed boots. A four-year-old can spot the butches, even if they aren't always so aware of it themselves. Queer author Trish Thomas says that she spent her pre-out years as a Stepford wife, drinking Pabst Blue Ribbon and watching *Wide World of Sports* on Sunday afternoons.

Cherchez la Femme.

Femme dykes are an entirely different breed. Long before "sheer lipstick" and "lesbian chic" became synonymous in the national media, lesbian dyna-femmes were expertly drawing on their eyeliner and completing eight-hour workdays in three-inch heels. Glamour dykes have functioned as some of our brightest Hollywood celebs and most notorious porn stars. How was anyone to know?

First, you have to look behind the lipstick. Fierce independence in a woman (and a decent manicure) is a dead giveaway. Look for that gal who doesn't seem to be standing by, leaning on, or fawning over a man. Compulsory heterosexuality is not so much about women desiring men as it is about women depending on them. Of course, lesbians *do* have a craving for soft curves and wet caresses, but lesbianism is just as much about living on our own terms as W-O-M-E-N.

Political inclinations are another dead giveaway. Find a radical feminist and you've got reasonable grounds to search for a lesbian. Yes, let's not be precious about this—you *can* scratch many a women's libber and find a ball-busting dyke. The Christian fundamentalist's bad dream contains a grain of truth: a feminist is bound to question conventional gender relations.

Only a lesbian could come up with a slogan like, "A woman needs a man like a fish needs a bicycle." Only dykes, especially the closeted ones, have the self-sacrificing zeal and energy to lead the fundraising for women's sports, fight for abortion rights, draw the line on sexual harassment, and mentor the next generation of female rocket scientists.

Why do dykes have five hundred ways to save the earth when most ordinary mortals only have fifty? It just goes to show that feminine sublimation goes a long way, especially when it's not directed towards the care and feeding of an ambitious husband. Lesbians have traditionally been shy and ambivalent about putting our own needs ahead of others. But we've also been women of extraordinary accomplishments, whether as pioneers like Margaret Mead or superstars like Martina and k.d. More commonly, we are the women who first volunteered at the AIDS hotline, the activists who started the battered women's shelter, the Amazons running the farm, protecting others from the storm. Auntie Em was a friend of Dorothy's, too, you know.

Sure, everyone wants to be a dyke now; they crave our freedom, guts, and knowing looks. When I saw a paparazzi photo of Axl Rose of Guns 'n' Roses wearing a "Nobody Knows I'm a Lesbian" tee-shirt, I didn't waste two seconds thinking about him. I looked a little closer at the picture because the woman who gave him that shirt must surely be in the background. Hey, did I say background? Pardon my disgusting pre–90's consciousness lapse. I'm sure the dyke was the smarty-pants snapping the shutter.

27

GAYDAR, OR IT TAKES ONE TO KNOW ONE

Adult Children of Family Values, or How Bush Lost the Election

IN LATE SUMMER of 1992, incumbent President George Bush and the Republican Party held a convention in Texas to proclaim their agenda for beating Clinton's Democratic ticket.

The Houston GOP get-together will be remembered forever for its Family Values Night, a Wednesday evening dedicated to insulting virtually everyone in America who didn't look like those attending the convention.

My local daily paper asked me to cover Family Values Night. They were too cheap to fly me to Houston, advising me instead to park my butt in front of C-SPAN for the evening. I'm forever grateful for their penny-pinching, since the ensuing evening of televised prejudice left me gasping on my knees in my own living room. Thankfully, I was safely home in Sodom-by-the-Sea.

I don't know where the Republican Party would be without "The Children." You know "The Children" are the whole reason that family values were even given one minute of Republican convention air time. "The Children" are the centerpiece of the Republican platform to turn this country around. As Governor John Ashcroft of Missouri said, if our children are not instilled with a moral purpose, "they will turn to the selfish gratification of drugs, promiscuity, rioting...and even mindless TV."

I closed my eyes for a moment to imagine such gluttony and realized that the hedonists passing across my mind's eye were not tiny tots or even petulant teenagers, but great big grown-ups.

When it comes to drugs, sex, violence, and even passing out cold in front of the television set, you can't beat the over-eighteen crowd. Adults—the kind who have had parents and grandparents (and even a public school teacher or two) to instill the basic Judeo-Christian work ethic from Day One—are the people who are falling through the thousands of black holes that separate George Bush's Points of

Light. All the GOP ticket had to say about them was that they obviously weren't raised right.

The Christian Right is at a loss to explain how millions of people who can recite Bible stories just as well as Pat Robertson are disaffected, degraded, or just plain down and out. Some of them had bootstraps, gave a good tug on them, and the straps broke. Others were born with beautiful boots, but preferring to feel the grass under their feet, threw them out.

It's a fact—when politicians don't have a clue about what's wrong with grown-ups in America, rich or poor, they turn to the subject of children: children's innocence, their malleability, their unmistakable victimhood.

Go ahead, get out the handkerchiefs, but before your eyes get red with anger or misty with sentiment, get a grip on this new code phrase. "The Children" doesn't mean the little ones who have to be in bed by nine—it means us, the big guys.

In the GOP family values tent, George and Babs are Mom and Dad, the Reagans are doting grandparents, and we voters are the babies. William Bennett, former drug czar and Education Secretary, spelled this out Wednesday night. "There are things children simply should not see," he said. But Bennett's not talking about your baby niece, he's talking about you, adult citizen.

Bush, after all, is the former chief of the CIA, an agency founded on the notion that there are many, many things the American public should not see. When we do catch a glimpse of a savings and loan scandal, or an opportunistic oil war, or a black man beaten into the ground by four white cops, we the people get the Simi Valley treatment: it's not us, it can't happen here, and it's business as usual.

In his nominating speech for Dan Quayle, Bennett wanted to be precise about his difference with Democrats. He declared, as happy as a biscuit, "We do not believe in handing out condoms to children."

Well, gee, Bill, what's your stand on handing out condoms to adulterous men over forty? How about housewives over twenty-five who put their careers on hold and their cookies in the oven? Should they have condoms? Should any American of voting age get disease prevention or birth control information?

The GOP is loathe to answer adult-size questions like these. In their view, The Children are the great unwashed of all ages—anyone from eight to eighty who can't buy his or her way out of a difficult situation. After all, giving out anything for free, let alone condoms, is gosh-darned communist.

The most moving message of Family Values Night in Houston came from an unheralded speaker, Mary Fisher, the daughter of presidential adviser and philanthropist Max Fisher. She is a personal friend of the Bushes. She is upper-middle-class and the blond mother of two preschoolers; she is also HIV-positive and president of the Family AIDS Network.

She wore a red ribbon on her lapel, a striking symbol of the Hollywood liberal elite, and she attacked ignorance and bigotry. She challenged the Republicans to get on the stick. She said she identified with poor black women and lonely gay men who were suffering from the same diagnosis as she. She scored a direct hit on the family values motif when she said, "We cannot praise the family and then ignore the virus that destroys it."

Fisher talked about her expectation that her children will be orphans. The TV camera panned the arena, picking up scores of bewildered, tear-stained faces, all women. She begged the party to put aside politics and make a sound policy.

That's when the atmosphere became all childlike again. Fisher never articulated what a sound policy might be. She pressed for parents to be "effective" educators of their children about AIDS, but how are moms and dads supposed to be "effective"? Would she advise her sons about condoms when they came of age? Would she go to their state-run school (that's the new post-Cold War euphemism for public schools) and deliver the same prime-time message she gave the GOP?

Fisher seemed to be hinting at a great deal of what the conservatives abhor. Her lines owed more to gay activism than to partisan politics. She must surely know that the right wing has no intention of creating an AIDS policy that doesn't put the blame on an "alternative lifestyle" for a disease that they repeatedly frame in moral terms: "What have you done to deserve this?"

Governor Pete Wilson of California appeared at the conference via satellite. We were told he'd been working day and night to solve our California budget crisis. I'm surprised he could find a moment to comb his hair for the camera. But he did, and his message was that Republicans are "compassionate conservatives." Dutiful paternalism struck again. Pete said that when a family has a budget problem, they sit down at the kitchen table and figure out which things are *non*essential—like a new car or refrigerator—versus what things are essential—like providing money for the kids' schooling.

I don't know what families Wilson is talking about, but my ancient refrigerator has been leaking for the past year, and my ten-year-old car is running on a prayer. At the moment, my toddler's day care costs as much as a one-bedroom apartment. I was kind of hoping I could send my daughter to a "state-run" school for free when she's old enough because I thought that was where my taxes were going!

Pete and George and Danny are like a lot of daddies that kids complain about these days—*they just don't get it.* Speaking for my generation, which is already old enough to know better, here's a message that any president, Democrat or Republican, should pay attention to: When it comes to hypocritical family values, as the GOP is so fond of saying, this will not stand.

31

ADULT
CHILDREN
OF FAMILY
VALUES

Puberty 2001

DURING THE FIRST decade of the twenty-first century, I will be going through puberty. Not my own of course, but my daughter's. If she's anything like I was, she'll be having sex for the very first time right around year 2005.

But wait a minute—I'm already talking like a twentieth-century relic. In the new age, I'd love to see my daughter recognize her sexual identity and need for pleasure long before her hymen is ritually torn. Don't get me wrong, I love old-fashioned ice cream sodas and old-fashioned sexual positions, but I hate the dreadful habit of saying "having sex" as if it equaled only penis/vagina intercourse.

When I masturbated as a young girl, I believed the devil was inside of me and that my clitoris was his seed. In fact, I was simply "having sex." When I practiced French kissing and no-translation-needed petting with my junior high school girlfriend, the pools of sweat we left in the bedroom were evidence that we were indeed "having sex." To this very day, I have never lain back after a decent pussy-licking, blow job, or bum-fucking, and sighed, "Are we having sex yet?"

It's not merely semantics I'm debating; it's a terrible prejudice we've inherited from our puritan forefathers—the first people in Western civilization to found a country with laws against adultery and fornication. The antifornication law is still on the books in nine states. Will it still be there when my daughter comes of age?

Sex in America has the dubious legacy of only being respectable when it is married to reproduction. Twentieth-century sex education has therefore consisted entirely of lectures on disease and pregnancy prevention. I remember my disappointment as a child to find that the main visual features of my first sex-ed book were diagrams of the sperm and the egg. How babies are born was not the foremost sex question on my eight-year-old mind.

I don't think I could have articulated it at the time, but what I really wondered was: Why do people wear clothes, and why is being nude sexy? What does an orgasm feel like? What is this place between my legs, and why does playing with Barbie turn me on?

I realized that sex education had become an oxymoron when I joined a speaker's bureau for local public high schools, created to talk to kids about gay and bisexual life. It was part of a program to counteract the antigay violence that had been spilling out of the school yard and into local parks and streets.

Our technique was to introduce ourselves, one man and one woman, to the Family Life class, and tell the kids how we discovered our sexual preferences—a thumbnail sexual history. They were free to ask any question they liked that afternoon, however gross or rude.

What struck me was that we, the queer guests, were the first people ever to talk about sex in the sex-education class. It would have been just as righteous for true-blue heterosexuals to step right up and explain how their first kisses felt, what it means to long for the opposite sex, and how they handle sexual risks and dilemmas.

Clearly, these issues were at the heart of every puberty-impaired student in the rooms I visited. Hormones are hell when you're a teenager; and being unable to understand what you're horny about, or why, leads to more problems than pimples or gay bashing.

I've been gearing up for the twenty-first century by instituting my own erotic literacy campaign. My daughter already knows the words for everything "down there," and by the time she's a ripe old adolescent I want her to know plenty more about her sexual desires and boundaries. I've been ready for the future of sex education ever since I put the sperm and egg diagrams aside in favor of Barbie. I'm sure my kid will be one step, and one century, ahead of me.

II. Reading Sex

ONE OF MY favorite books about feminism and sex is Carole Vance's *Pleasure and Danger.* The title was a winner, inspired by the double standard women face when they pursue their own sexual adventures.

If I did a sequel to *Pleasure and Danger,* exploring another facet of the erotic dialectic, I might call it *Pleasure and Stupidity,* or *Hot Sex and Dumb Blondes.*

In the American arts community, when authors, musicians, or actors get explicit about sexuality, we assume they have lost their marbles. Only vacant, low-IQ people think about sex all the time, right? It's superficial, it's for lower species, it's for dilettantes who don't care or even realize that people are starving in India. It's interesting that people in other countries like India, starving or not, don't have such a condescending attitude toward Eros.

It works the other way, too. People who are thought to be intelligent or deep are presumed to have terribly boring sex lives. The public is unsettled when Einstein's torrid love letters are revealed—how unscientific of him! Maybe he wasn't such a genius after all....

Joe DiMaggio and Marilyn Monroe made sense, Marilyn Monroe and Arthur Miller did not. It is as if the brains and the body are destined to cancel each other out.

One day I went to the beach with a journalist who said to me, "I don't mean to insult you...it's hard to say this without being patronizing...you'll probably take this the wrong way...but I was really surprised that you write so well." He considered me an anomaly, a literate pornographer.

I'd like to bend the stick in the other direction a little, and suggest that the artists who take the deepest and most provocative looks at sexuality are actually the movers and shakers of our time—even likely to have a touch of genius.

The following essays critique the work of writers and artists whose integrity has come into question because of their sexual interests. Author Nicholson Baker ("Fermata-cize Me!" and "Sex and the Single Reader") is thought by dozens of his peers to have "ruined his career" because he stopped writing about elevator rides and started writing about climaxes. Madonna ("A Pornographic Girl") is an entertainer whose judgment is constantly called into question because of her reputation as a sex maniac. Other girl singers may be quantifiably dumber than Madonna, but because they don't take their clothes off, their intelligence doesn't come under such scrutiny. Personally, I think the smartest thing smart people can do is take off their clothes.

Stephen King ("Tie Me Up, Bog Me Down") doesn't suffer from accusations that he's going soft in the head because of the eroticism of his recent horror writing. That's because he kills all his kinky characters. Likewise, Dr. Ruth, a sex expert and celebrity ("She Knows What She Likes"), enhances her intellectual reputation by heaping on irreverent humor and disdain for all things erotic. Condoms? Yes. "Unsafe" wet dreams? No. Although she is a sexual celebrity, we have a hard time imagining her having sex, and it's not because of her age, it's her attitude.

Finally, in "Femmchismo," I explore the very smart literary possibilities that could occur when women reject the feminine masquerade of innocence in favor of sexual decisiveness and even conceit.

It may be tough on folks to imagine that one can have a fierce mind and a great sex life to boot. If that incites envy, too bad—envy's exactly where all the criticism and denial come from. I'd rather search my mind and body together for divine inspiration.

Femmchismo

WHEN I FIRST started teaching women's erotic writing classes in 1989, I didn't know who would show up. After all, who hasn't written—in her diary, or on the back of a matchbook—at least a few sweaty words, a love poem, a passionate letter?

But teaching a class to women writers on the art of sensual writing showed me that something more was afloat than the inalienable right to serenade one's lover. Women's erotica, as it has come to be called, is a new genre of literature—fiction that illustrates the very real changes that have occurred in women's sexual interests and desires.

Women are hungry—no, ravenous—for sexual knowledge and erotic inspiration. They are offended by notions of romance that exclude sexual satisfaction or play innocent; indeed, it's no surprise when a woman sings a hit song called "What's Love Got to Do with It?" We have a new understanding about our bodies' sexual responses.

We experience sex in and out of all the traditions of love, commitment, marriage, and child rearing. We make love with men and women, sometimes in fantasy, sometimes in real life. Sometimes we are men in our sexual imaginations. We take in the sexual signs of our times—X-rated home video, AIDS awareness, G-spot ejaculations, condoms, marriage burn-out, date rape, single motherhood, lesbian visibility, vibrator availability. We take in the realities of sex in our era and we insist on including these slices of real life in our erotica; indeed, we delight in it.

I like to play a game in my erotica classroom. I ask everyone to write a beginning erotic sentence, something easy like, "She touched her clit."

"Now keep on going," I say, "and do it in the style of a plain-brown-wrapper novel, the kind of book you'd find in the back of the sleaziest store in town."

Two minutes later I tell them to stop. "Now switch," I say, "and start writing as if this were a free verse, uninhibited love poem that you wrote on the cliffs of Big Sur." Then I have them switch again, two minutes later, to a supermarket bodice-ripper: "Me, Rhett; you, Scarlett." Switch again to a '50s beatnik ultra-hip cigarette-after-the-screw style. No matter how unsophisticated the writer, each student has had some glancing experience with each of the styles I ask them to imitate.

Finally, I ask them to end their stories in one last genre. "Finish your story in a 'women's erotica' style," I tell them. And they jump right in. No one asks me anymore, "What are you talking about?" Despite the continual media complaint that no one knows what women want, apparently women do have a collective sense of what they expect out of a sexy story, and it's so well known that I can even ask my students to give me a quick treatment of it.

I used to have one impeccable standard for what made an erotic story female-centered: the woman comes. This single concept is so rare in traditional erotica that it overwhelms every other feminine consideration. Of course we've all read stories where a woman is overwhelmed with the size of her lover's penis, she screams his name and clutches his breast—but how many times do you actually get a her-point-of-view orgasm? We read about how he sees her responding to him, but we don't see inside her explosion. I still believe a woman's climax makes a good bottom line for women's erotica. But now I have other angles to consider. There are other aspects of women's literary libidos that show their colors just as brilliantly as any hot pink orgasm.

I call the primary signal of the burgeoning women's erotica movement "femmchismo." This is exactly what it sounds like: the aggressive, seductive, and very hungry sexual ego of a woman. Like machismo, it embodies an erotic arrogance; for women, it's clear this is a long overdue form of conceit. Femmchismo has been a well-kept secret. Women have always talked among themselves in classic pajama-party bravado about their awareness of their sexual power and talent. Sometimes this boasting takes the form of dubious self-effacement. Typically, a woman would not brag openly about having a big ass the way a man might boast of his big cock—but she gets her message across, talking about what a trial it is to be the object of such enormous desire.

Femmchismo draws both on a woman's desirability—the excitement she creates by simply "being" there—and on her sexual talents to influence and make love to her intended subject.

Certainly the stereotype of the female predator is not new: the spider, the manipulator, the schemer. The sex-negative caricature of woman's sexual aggression is that she is evil and that she seeks destruction and castration, not an orgasm. Her scheme of sexual wiles is to procure something other than sex. What's new in women's erotica is that, when women describe their sexual courage and pride, erotic satisfaction is their explicit goal.

To be sexually adventurous for her own sake, to feel her desire and to direct it for ultimate satisfaction—yes, this is femmchismo, and don't be surprised if its hard little clit comes rubbing up against your leg—purring, of course. Femmchismo is emphatically not about falling in love, or about "the very first time." It's about the value of a unique sexual experience: desire empowered by action.

When feminists and writers first started discussing the future of women's erotica, there was a call for a new woman-centered language, a modern vocabulary to discuss women's sexual feelings. As an editor, I find that the language is there—at the tips of our tongues. What is harder than imagining the words is saying them out loud.

Street vocabulary is easily possessed by women who find no embarrassment in the shape of erotic women's language. Street slang is just as your mother taught you: absolutely unladylike. But how many "ladies" under sixty haven't said "fuck" by now, either in anger or passion? What women have to cope with in employing four-letter words is not that they aren't suited to us. They suit us just fine when we aren't afraid of being shushed by some double standard of judgment.

Obscene words are powerful and forceful; that's why they are deemed unsuitable for ladies—who are weak and delicate. When we have indelicate sexual feelings, we get a little choked up; there don't seem to be ladies' words for lustful emotions. "Ladies" don't lust. But real women do, and it's perfectly appropriate for us to use strong language when the situation calls for it.

Most disputes over erotic language center on trying to find perfect alternatives to certain words. Is *vagina* too medical or too clinical? Is *cunt* too mean? I think we're splitting hairs in the wrong direction over such quests for the ideal synonyms. What's really missing in our erotic language are descriptions of women's arousal—from the first flush of desire and wetness, to the climactic loss of control, to the multiple sensations after orgasm.

Lesbian erotica has been the fastest changing and most controversial aspect of the bloom in women's erotica. Lesbian sex stories have been around forever, but they typically were not written by or for lesbians. They were stories about breaking taboo, about the sexual possibilities of manlessness. They were more about the absent men than they were about the present women.

When lesbians began to speak for themselves erotically, it was often in the context of coming-out stories—women discovering they liked other women. Self-discovery is the key to the sexual excitement in a coming-out scenario; yet for a woman of any lesbian experience, the first sexual encounter is unlikely to be the most satisfying and revealing experience she'll ever have with another woman. Losing one's virginity may be a big deal, but it's rarely the best sex a woman will ever have.

What's new in the '90s are lesbian characters who are grown-ups—women who not only desire and love other women, but also have the same sophisticated and diverse sexual tastes as heterosexual females. In the past, lesbian protagonists were ingenues, whether they were fifteen or forty, questioning their sexuality, yearning for the security of knowing themselves. The content of new lesbian literature presents heroines who are nobody's fools, whose lesbianism is a matter of course.

So much of contemporary women's fiction is outrageous simply because it is not stereotypical. While daytime talk shows regale us with the spectacle of "Black Lesbians" or "Lesbian Moms Who Like Porn," the new lesbian erotic literature is an understated command to get over it. Not only is there a lesbian under every bed, but she comes in every color, lifestyle, and political opinion.

The first revolution in lesbian erotic literature was writing from the lesbian point of view. That seems obvious and overdue enough to understand immediately. But the second revolution in lesbian erotica is not really about lesbianism per se. It's about gender-bending and the vicarious experience of erotically placing yourself in another's shoes.

Genderbending is a complete departure from the closely held myth that lesbians are utterly divorced from any kind of vicarious masculine appreciation. Lesbian purity has been like the last white dress anybody could find to cover up the fact that sexual imaginations wander everywhere. Just because a woman has no interest in a relationship with a man doesn't mean that she might not fantasize about sex with a man, or perhaps imagine being a man. Our fantasies, like our nightly dreams, are not compromised in the least by who we live with and love in the real world.

More than any other group of writers, lesbian erotic writers have grabbed genderbending by the genitals and taken the whole spectrum of masculine/feminine eroticism by storm. Radical lesbian sex writers took one of porn's most common questions and turned it upside down: Why do so many men like to watch lesbian sex? The hip lesbian answer is, "Because everybody can and does fantasize about anybody and anything they please."

When an ostensibly heterosexual woman writes of her desire for a man, she can also defy traditional roles. It's not unusual at all to find a story where the woman dominates her male lover, or the man acts as her servant. This fantasy has been seen many times, mainly because it's such a popular turn-on for men.

The rare female twist to this role reversal is where the woman not only takes control, but also takes on a man's feelings and prerogatives—which have less to do with domination and more to do with the masculine world. In one of my favorite stories, "Taking Him on a Sunday Afternoon," author Magenta Michaels describes how a wife turns the tables on her husband:

> *He clamps up to prevent me from rubbing him there, but aggression has risen in me and I press on, massaging a moistened finger at his entrance. It's slick there and I can imagine the smell, which excites me; I know that he's concerned about the smell, too—how I'll find him—and this excites me even more.*

This phrase, "how I'll find him," epitomizes the role reversal. Traditionally, it is women who "get found," ladies who worry about what they smell like, and men who relish this vulnerability.

Sometimes women subvert male sexual excitement by making their own submission almost, but not quite, impossible. They thrive on exuding as well as seeking masculine energy. It's like a Valkyrie demanding her due. The language that new women pornographers seek is not about love, at least not the Valentine card love that women have long believed was the greatest literary expectation of our passion. Women are approaching a new lover's language today, a roar that comes straight out of our undulating bellies.

A Pornographic Girl: Madonna's *Sex*

WHEN MADONNA PUBLISHED her first "dirty" book, I was first in line to purchase a fifty-dollar copy. Like most of the baby-boomer, thirty-something audience targeted by Madonna's *Sex*, I received a typical little girl's education about sex, and it went something like this:

(1) Girls don't know very much about sex, and they don't need to know more.

(2) Girls need love, not sex.

(3) Don't expect to come.

I know that Madonna was brought up this very same way.

In our childhood, men were typically described as inherently aggressive, naturally promiscuous and objectifying, exclusively genitally focused, prone to sexual addictions and dangerous pornographic masturbation, and in general needing to be contained so that their active pursuit of sexuality wouldn't be a public menace.

Women, on the other hand, were lauded for our inherently sexual gentility and monogamous nature; our desire was equated with romantic love, our sex with a nurturing, non-genitally focused sensuality. Sexual pleasure and liberation were absolutely not priorities for women. Finally, women never used, produced, or enjoyed pornography.

And if you believe any of the above, I've got a great little piece of property to show you on Love Canal....

The early women's liberation movement threw these notions in the trash, and sooner than you could say "Eat my clit," women were revealing their sexual appetites in unprecedented numbers. In a vulva-shaped nutshell, the message was: find your clit, learn to create your orgasm, express your sexual curiosity to its fullest, and don't let anyone, especially any man, tell you how to get off.

During my years as a sex activist, introducing women to the words that describe our sexual lives, to the pictures of our bodies and desires, to the confidence of hearing other women's common and kinky sexual experiences—well, there's been no turning back. Sexually, there is nothing new under the sun. But there are still so many shadows, and it has been the talking and writing and revealing that have cast us into the light.

Madonna's best intentions, however, were scorned from coast to coast.

So what was so bad about *Sex?*

Thousands of people had a ready answer, thousands who never touched the mylar bag o'erotica called *Sex* that pop celebrity Madonna fashioned to illustrate her sexual fantasies. The indignant consumer sounded the battle cry: "I will not buy this book. I *refuse.*"

It was a particularly American outrage, and it began with an apparently innocent penny-pinching reproach: This book costs too much. Who would pay fifty dollars for a book?

The people who would not pay fifty dollars for a book were the very group that was trashing *Sex* as they left trendy cafés with sixty-dollar margarita bills; they were the ones who sniffed at the idea of erotica but spent forty dollars on cat calendars at Barnes and Noble; they were the people who didn't buy hard-cover books all year—but Nintendo owns their MasterCards.

Face it, the market for Madonna's book was never intended to be teenagers with lousy allowances, or the unemployed monitoring their January heating bills. This was a book for yuppies, art book fanciers, and erotica enthusiasts, all of whom are known to blow money on items both extremely personal and of questionable taste.

The other reason for not buying *Sex* was Celebrity Nausea. We gagged on Hillary Rodham Clinton's cookies, we didn't give a damn if Drew Barrymore got married, and if one more adult child of Ronald Reagan wrote an autobiography we were going to hurl. There's something to be said for the ennui and exasperation we feel when fifteen-minute celebrities publish the meager facts of their lives.

But with Madonna, the subject at hand elicited something a little closer to envy—many of us wouldn't have minded having budgets to illustrate our sexual imaginations. Some artists were in a state of shock over the news that Madonna had taken the substance of their cutting-edge erotic *tour de force* and turned it into profitable shelf space at Crown Books. I sympathized with those unheralded sex pioneers, because they're my comrades. But we were no different from some Harlem vogue diva watching MTV with his mouth hanging open at Madonna's Hollywood-ization of his original achievement.

Labeling the book a rip-off, either financial or artistic, does not warrant the bile that came from the lips of the media and man-on-the-street critics. What was hated about *Sex* was that it was "tawdry," "adolescent," "violent," and "kinky." Stripped of those pejoratives, the criticism's essence was an attack on the book's single-minded sexual premise. It was prima facie S-E-X that offended them—and hold onto your Kinsey Institute report—because sexual fantasies, whether they be Madonna's or anyone else's, are based on taboos, infantile (not to mention adolescent) memories, and repressed desires which are often similar in sensation to fear and anger. Welcome to the world of the sexual unconscious.

The reputable side of erotica is tenderness and sensuality, a rapport between flesh and nature. This is well represented in Madonna's book. She is a love child, just a skip away from flower power. Many of her book's images are filled with romance, gentleness, and humor—in fact, those pictures are the most affecting images in the book. A picture of Madonna applying lipstick to her boy lover's lips is more poignant in its delicacy than any shock from its genderbending insinuations. Madonna's face on a pillow in the dark, her thumb to her mouth and eyes beginning to tear, evokes a lonely ache that is undeniable. Then there's Madonna's famous crotch, her mound of Venus arched in a beachball spray of water, her dark pubic curls so luscious and different from her blonde wigginess.

Madonna is at her best in vanilla, at least through photographer Stephen Meisel's approximation. In total though, Madonna takes on the *Penthouse Letter* portfolio of fantasies—every naughty thought on America's mind: black/white relations, Daddy's little girl, older seductress, crossdressing, group sex, doggie sex, exhibitionism, and non-specific wantonness. True, her take on it all is not original, her photographer's eye is not transcendent.

Yet upon publication the images were still provocative, still had the power to affect us, simply because they were *her* Genuine Article. We, the audience, were completely unaccustomed to anyone's being straightforward about what they like in bed.

Let's be candid: the reason there was a public outcry about *Sex* is that Americans don't think sex should be discussed in the light of day. Look at the polls on homosexuality. When it comes to what you do when the lights are out, no one gives a damn. A clandestine act of sodomy is far, far preferable to two men kissing in the park.

Americans, and our puritanical ancestors, the British, love nothing so much as to put down sex for being sexual. Nothing elevates one's standing like a carefully arch quote that rains on the erotic parade. It's ever so clever to say what you *don't* like, and completely *outré* to say what you *do*.

The biggest, most profound problem with Madonna's sexual encyclopedia (aside from the wretched binding job) was that it was produced with a set of instructions straight from the censor's little black book. Madonna was given a green light from her publisher, Time Warner, as long as she refrained from pictures with penetration, explicit genitalia, sex with animals, and sex with children. This is a laundry list accepted by every legitimate publisher in the country, but what kind of sense does it make? What on earth do those four no-nos have to do with each other?

Madonna's writing is far more revealing than the photographs. We learn from her "diary entries" that she is a typical red-blooded American girl; she likes getting her pussy licked almost better than anything. When being fucked, she manipulates her clitoris to reach orgasm, and the only position where she takes a hands-off approach is on top. She likes to wake up and feel her lover's erection at her back. She's not fond of blow jobs, but she's impressed to see one expertly performed. She speaks as highly of masturbation as Shere Hite. She is not ashamed of her genitals, and she treasures her pussy as a source of life and pleasure.

But none of this basic introduction to women's sexual liberation is illustrated in her book. We never see Madonna masturbate, or have intercourse, let alone have an orgasm. We never witness any of the models making the kind of faces that reveal sexual ecstasy, because they never did the slightest thing that would make them lose control.

Instead of going all the way, we get kinky foreplay. The most controversial photos in Madonna's book are sadomasochistic. Her accompanying words are vulnerable and thoughtful about this notoriously misunderstood topic. But the pictures are as static as a Velcro release on a leather sling. S/M erotica in this county is permitted by law to show fetish, bondage, or any style of whipping—this is considered R-rated and acceptable. The line we are not supposed to cross is to *combine* genital sexuality with these same images—an act so bold as to force the artist/producer into a underground and illegal oblivion. To the uninitiated, this means that S/M in Madonna's book and elsewhere looks like a blackened kitchen demonstration. It's completely diabolical. If the point in getting spanked is to get off, then why do we never see the *getting off* part?

Somebody, and I wish it could be a star with Madonna's power, needs to make a break with the standard obscenity code in this country, which insists that the most elemental (not to mention vanilla) sexual acts cannot be depicted because they are too dirty. If there's nothing disgusting about a woman's vulva, then why can't we see a picture of it without pornographic accusations? If making love is where love and ecstasy and babies come from, then what kind of absurd, hateful laws do we have that forbid its artistic portrayal?

Madonna searched desperately for a printer in the United States. One finally came through, but did not allow its name to be used in connection with the book. It tickled me to see that even Miss Invincible was faced with the problem every two-bit pornographer faces: no one turns on their press for dirty pictures. The commercial pornography industry survives in this country only because it bought and built its own printing plants.

In the same spirit, Madonna "bought" the right to publish a book like this. The wealthy have always had the ultimate access to freedom of speech, but few of them stuck their necks out as she did. What was missing in all the tirades about Madonna's mediocrity was that this book is by far her most serious work to date, both in her execution and her confrontation with the status quo. Her songs are tunes with a good beat that you can dance to. Her movie appearances have been embarrassing eighty percent of the time. Her politics, though, are Madonna's most original strength. She possesses the outspoken feminist idealism and compassionate philanthropy that has made liberal heroines out of Susan Sarandon, Whoopi Goldberg, and Jane Fonda. The popularity they enjoy with the politically correct has eluded Madonna for one reason only: she is a "sex maniac." And being a very public and willing sex maniac is the most original, radical, and courageous thing that Madonna Ciccone has ever done.

Sex and the Single Reader

IT WAS A stroke of genius. A stroke-book of genius, in fact. The reviewer's copy of *VOX* arrived: a slim volume wrapped in a plain brown paper wrapper, with a large black "X" stamped on the lower right-hand corner. One would not open a cover like this without inviting the taint of perversion. It was truly racy.

On the back of the plain brown wrapper another few letters appeared, spelling out "Random House." And here the publisher's real wit showed, because can you imagine Random House printing fifty thousand copies of a porn novel? What a hoot! But it is not a hoot—it is Faux Porn.

Faux Porn has become very, very big. The label "erotica" is so vague as to try one's patience, and the title "pornography" is criminalized. But this new genre, called "sexual candor" in the most sophisticated circles, is about to reach deep inside your ding-a-ling-ling and make a reader out of you.

All the serious young literati are in on it. When I read that Naomi Wolf, author of the feminist fashion exposé *The Beauty Myth,* had received a $500,000 advance for her *Lolita*-like, somewhat autobiographical tale of "sexual candor," I nearly croaked. I have not had the pleasure, you see, of being called "sexually candid." The words "trash," "perverted," and "obscene" have all been used to describe my books (in one case, women's erotic short stories, in the other, sex-filled lesbian essays). My work has been banned in South Africa, New Zealand, Canada and Madison, Wisconsin. What's the difference between mine and theirs? Obviously it is just a matter of marketing—not to mention connections. I am jealous. I am steaming.

So as an apple-pie pornographer with nothing to hide, I blistered when Nicholson Baker, the author of *VOX,* was interviewed in *Vanity Fair.* He said that he always wanted to be a pornographer when he grew up. What a little charmer! This was right after *Vanity Fair* said he was the best writer of our generation and threw in a comparison to Hemingway for good measure. I was pissed. Nicholson Baker was trifling with a serious issue here. I resolved to call Mr. Next Big Thing and put him to the test.

Nick Baker is so nice on the phone that it took all my triple X-rated strength to maintain a moral fury. "I don't believe that you would really like to be a pornographer," I told him. "If you were a porn writer, no one would know who you were. Your work would be published under a pseudonym or anonymously. If exposed, you could be tried in any court and found guilty of the mysterious crime of obscenity. You would be put in jail, your house seized. Your children would be taken away from you.

"I don't believe you want to be a pornographer," I choked, "because you have no idea what it means to be ostracized for your sexual beliefs."

"Well, that's a legitimate outrage," Baker replied. "I do think there was a tad of smirkiness about it [*VOX*]. But on the other hand, it did work: people's interest was piqued."

His graceful concession notwithstanding, I pressed him further. Here is a man who not only was the packaging phenomenon of 1992, he also wrote a book which consists entirely of a phone-sex conversation between a man and a woman on opposite coasts. They find each other through a commercial 900 party line and switch over to a private line for a more intimate conversation.

But what follows is not a beat-the-clock jack-off contest between the two. They discuss their erotic fantasies and experiences patiently, even shyly. Baker's style is famous for artful digression. His best known book before this was *Mezzanine*, a hundred-page ditty that consists entirely of a man taking an office break to buy a pair of shoelaces. True to form, his phone-sex characters get distracted at the drop of a hat, away from their erotic momentum and into what they ate for lunch.

"You're a terrible tease," I told Baker. "You brought me wobbling to the brink several times, and…"

"No payoff, huh?" he interrupted.

"Exactly: the classic prick-tease in book form. Here, here's the worst example—" I thumbed to the scene that had made me throw the book down on the floor. "Page 146!" I announced, "Let me read it to you:

"And it was exactly what I wanted, and it started to feel so
good, and I said so and suddenly he started stroking himself

incredibly fast, it was this blur, like a sewing machine, and he produced this major jet of sperm at a diagonal right into the circular spray of the water, so that it fought against all the drops and was sort of torn apart by them, and he was clamping my leg, my smooth leg, extremely tight with those perfectly water-groomed thighs, and I shifted adroitly so that the poached sperm and hot-water runoff wouldn't pour directly into me and possibly cause trouble, but so that it still poured over me. And then he took the showerhead again, and still holding his cock, and still clamping my knee very tight, he sprayed slowly across my hand and my thighs very close with the water until I closed my eyes and came, imagining I was in front of a circus audience. So that was very nice."

"God of mercy, I am so jealous!"

"Don't be," she said. "I think my offhand talk of yeast unnerved him…"

I paused dramatically, wondering if Baker had heard his own Faux Porn read back to him. "I can't believe you blew off the end of that fantasy to bring up a *yeast infection!*" I yelled. "Who wants an orgasm that ends with, 'So that was very nice'?!"

"I wasn't actively trying to frustrate the reader," Nick said. "I wanted a realistic conversational texture. I wanted the characters to entertain each other, by teasing, dropping the thread provocatively. The most graphic moments are not necessarily in your private loops. It's some other moment. It's out of order, and especially as you get close to orgasm, the dishevelment, the memories get shuffled. I tried to capture that."

Memories and dishevelment are fine, I told him, but leaving your reader with a case of blue balls or an aching clit is not. At a certain point, he has to drop the self-consciousness, get down on the floor, and grind like anyone else.

I flipped to the end of the book where our two lovers finally do get off. "This was the most boring scene of all," I said. "After the fantasy with the painters? The Victoria's Secret warehouse? The olive oil scene?"

"I got such different Nielsen numbers for the different scenes," Baker said. "Some people thought the best was the last."

"The last scene could have made it if you hadn't inserted your little 'Johnny-on-the-thesaurus' touches," I railed. "Now look at this paragraph:

"I'd take one last lick on your pussy and then I'd straighten up, and I'd still be cupping your ass in my hands, and you'd be completely visible by now, wide open, and sopping wet, and I'd take my cock in one hand and kind of vibrate it over your clit, and you'd slide your hands down and hold your lips apart with your fingers, and then I'd push my cock down and I'd feel how hot you were and I'd have to slide myself slowly all the way in, and then I'd pull almost all the way out again and slide in, into that nice nasturtium..."

"Now, Nick, why would I want to hear about 'nice nasturtiums' at a time like this?" I said.

"I love that word!" Nick cried. "I am more proud of that word than anything else in the scene!"

"I know, it's lovely," I said. "It's lyrical. But it interrupted my path of arousal, my identification with the speaker, and reminded me of you, the author, sticking his precious 'best writer of our generation' vocabulary in. When I'm heading down the final ramp at the orgasm factory, there are no nasturtiums, Nick. There are only pistons."

"But they are down there," Nick said. "They are, they're like a bolt from heaven. The vocabulary illuminates the guy's conversation, it jostles what is happening...It was a moment of triumph!"

Clearly, this novel is a love child. And as if I were Linus on the eve of Halloween, I concluded that the author is a sincere pumpkin, and despite his timidity, a bit of a risk taker. Baker is quite right that his book gives many different readings on the arouse-o-meter. I passed my copy around to five friends and got wildly varied reviews from each of them. Women gave it higher ratings than men.

Ironically, *VOX* is the most overtly feminist sex novel that anyone has attempted in years. I say that because the female character is erotically on a par with her male partner. She is articulate, lusty, and supplied with normal female caution—but just as normally, with feminine curiosity and desire.

The characters also embody the feminist ambivalence concerning sexual taboos, violence, and power quotients. Compared, let's say, to Anne Rice's erotic novels, published under her pseudonym A.N. Roquelaure (*Beauty's Punishment*, etc.), Baker is more style-conscious and wholesome. But Rice's gender-blender S/M fantasia will burn out your vibrator faster.

When I read the ad copy on the back cover of *VOX*—"The most sexually provocative novel of our time!"—I thought, "I don't think so."

Nevertheless, Baker is the first male erotic novelist whose ancestors are the pioneers of the women's erotic movement. This book could not have been written before them. This is an important marker. Especially coming as it does from a major publisher. It's not a bodice-ripper or a Palm Beach exposé, not a Dworkinesque tract against porn that really is pornographic, but a genuine erotic story for grown-ups. I don't think it goes far enough—I warned Baker he would get only a "half-erect" rating from me—but at least it's in the ballpark.

"What are you wearing?" the male character asks his phone date in the first line of the book.

"A white shirt," she says, "with little white stars, green and black stars, and black pants, and socks the color of the green stars, and a pair of black sneakers I got for nine dollars."

If nothing else, Baker has demystified phone sex. I found myself asking the same question, "What are you wearing?" to every person I talked to on the phone for a week. Usually I got the nine-dollar-sneakers-type answers, although some disheveled surprises leapt from the receiver.

"So what are you wearing right now?" I asked Nicholson Baker.

He changed the subject.

"Thank you for complicating my life so gracefully," he said. "It's probably good for me to have one critic attacking me from the left."

"I'm not kidding, Nick," I said. "I won't hang up until you tell me what you're wearing." A *VOX*-like silence hung over the line.

"Well," he finally replied, "I have a Smith and Hawkins' Santa Rosa plum-colored cap on my knee...and that's all I'm going to tell you."

What did I tell you about this guy? A tease. If you see him on tour and he refuses to read or talk dirty, don't let him get away with it. Sexual candor, and even Faux Porn, demand nothing less.

Tie Me Up, Bog Me Down

WHAT HAS STEPHEN King got against bondage? B-O-N-D-A-G-E, the "ohh-baby" kind, not the "metaphor for human suffering" kind, is the use of restraint in erotic foreplay. It is also the fetish and villain of King's best-seller, *Gerald's Game*. Gerald's fascination with tying up his wife, Jessie, is the kinky side trip of an otherwise uptight and upscale lawyer, and it leads to his own accidental death in the first twenty pages. But the trauma inflicted on Jessie has larger and more horrific consequences.

Gerald's Game is an ugly stereotype about how sexual desire leads men into the blackest of holes. Although bondage is the erotic focus of the plot, it is probably too much to imagine that King has a special grudge against this particular kind of sex. The story is much more ordinary: a simple tale of a woman victimized by male lust. The Snidely Whiplash figure of yore need not tie Fair Nell to the railroad tracks—or the bedframe; he can leave her hanging from a cliff in any number of ways.

No one hears Jessie as she screams, alone in her summer cottage after everyone has gone home for autumn. Her husband had handcuffed her to the bedposts, ready for his sport, but she kicked him in the balls—her first act of defiance in years—and he suffered a heart attack that killed him on the spot.

We are accustomed to women sickened by men's fantasies; we are familiar with the boor who cannot hear his lover's entreaties to STOP STOP STOP. The most insightful part of King's whole book is the quotation he uses to preface his story, a line from Somerset Maugham's "Rain": "[Sadie] gathered herself together. No one could describe the scorn of her expression or the contemptuous hatred she put into her answer. 'You men! You filthy pigs! You're all the same, all of you. Pigs! Pigs!' " If this is how a male author characterizes his morality, whether in sincere self-loathing or bemused sarcasm, then nothing will ever evolve in literature as it has in real life, and women will as surely be victims as men will be devils.

Devilish King has one particularly famous signature: the gross part. Gerald's body lies sprawled on the floor, gnawed on by a stray dog, while our heroine lies cuffed to the bed, dying of thirst, floating in and out of consciousness. She relives not only her hapless marriage, but also her disturbing relationship with her father. Jessie gets put through the wringer (or shall we say the handcuff), and of course, since this is a best-seller, she eventually triumphs over adversity.

Long before the feminist therapy movement created labels like "incest survivor" and "pornography victim," women were sacrificial lambs for men's assumed uncontrollable and callous sexual behavior. When the motto "Pornography causes violence against women" first leapt from feminist lips, we were carefully retracing a much older tradition: sex will lead to women's ruin. A heroine cannot be too sexually sophisticated or hungry without suffering the punishment of being damned as a whore.

King's novel is a pyramid of such clichés, rooted in the days when a woman's sexuality was no more than her reproductive essence, her security blanket. Dead Gerald is certainly a pig, a classic insensitive white male lawyer. Whatever innocence or charm he had as a young man has been replaced by his hollow status-searching. "Selling out" has perverted him; he needs girlie mags and metal restraints to get him hard and get him off.

Lie Number One: When a man sells his soul to the corporation, he can't enjoy vanilla sex anymore.

I've got news for you: lots of Really Big Sellouts enjoy the missionary position best of all—and, on the other hand, there are plenty of tender, poetic vegetarians who get off on *Penthouse Letters* and black Velcro restraints.

Jessie is neither a sellout nor a radical. She's a victim who only fights back when faced with death. To summon the courage to get herself out of this mess, she has to come clean about her childhood sexual experience with her father. Since she is alone except for the man-eating Labrador, she speaks only to the two competing voices inside her head. Each one appears in italics and, like a little angel and devil, they tug on Jessie's conscience.

The "Goodwife"—the doubtful timid woman who presumably lives in every woman's head—tells Jessie that what happened to her is her own fault, to accept the inevitable; she should accept piety instead of power.

The opposing voice is "Ruth," a former college roommate of Jessie's, the no-nonsense feminist who is going to champion Jessie out of her hellhole. Ruth is the perfect militant who has no patience for the secrets of a dysfunctional family, no time for self-effacing denial.

But Ruth lacks one crucial aspect of the liberated woman: her voice never expresses the cry of female sexual self-determination. She pounces on Gerald's white-collar machismo, she savages Jessie's father. But Ruth never speaks out about what Jessie might want for her own sexual satisfaction. Ruth, the voice of common sense and dignity, lacks a libido.

King is an architect of female protectionism playing hard and fast under feminist rhetoric. Men, exemplified by Daddy and Husband, are pretentious sexual brutes who are impossible to identify with. We hear over and over again how much Jessie loved her dad, but we, the readers, never love him, not for a moment. The second he reaches his hand between her thighs is as predictable as it is creepy. When he comes in his pants from clumsily clutching his daughter to his lap, the reader gets the full horror story of his spilled seed, the awful stain that won't go away.

Why is semen—more than blood, pus, and sewage put together— the most grotesque bodily fluid in American literature? The King James Bible seems to be our companion reader to every Stephen King novel.

Many women and men have talked about their incest experiences from a complex, i.e. realistic, point of view. Their adult sexual fantasies and lives run the gamut from those who avoid sex altogether to those who enjoy all manner of sex, romantic or kinky.

Lie Number Two: Incest automatically turns children into queers, celibates, or masochistic adults.

No one is predisposed to S/M, or any other sexual desire or fetish, as a result of incest. Today, in liberal circles, no one believes the myth that ugly childhood experiences turn kids into homosexuals. But all the old bugaboos about the causes and effects of homosexuality, so popular before the gay rights movement, are now applied wholesale to less understood sexual preferences like bondage.

Over her protests, Gerald reminds his wife that the first time he tied her up with silk scarves, she loved it, she came so hard it almost broke the bed. Was this the proof I longed for—that Jessie had her own erotic gunpowder to be dealt with? Oh, no, the hidden voices in Jessie's head quickly explain. Jessie only enjoyed it the first time because she was able to give up responsibility, just like she longed to give up responsibility for her guilty conscience over "letting" her dad touch her.

Chalk up another one to the puritan army. When did letting go of responsibility in sex become a psychological crime? Is orgasm's sweet relief only a reminder of what pigs and victims we really are?

I want to know the real reason that Jessie came the first time she was tied up—and never again. Her strong sexual episodes seem infrequent, yet revolutionary. When she finally frees herself and gets up to quench her thirst at the end, "she thought she would never again experience anything as deeply satisfying as those first few swallows of cold water from the gushing tap; and in all her previous experience, only her first orgasm came close to rivaling that moment." Naturally, there's not another word said about this extraordinary memory.

It is not incongruous that Jessie might enjoy bondage over and over again with a more empathetic partner. Her orgasms as a mature woman might be the most powerful in her life if she had a lover who at least had a clue when enough was enough.

But men never know when enough is enough, right? Women have to take special courses in how to say no, because men are biologically incapable of...what? Self-discipline? Patience? Control? Men seem so good at those things in every other aspect of life. It's curious that, in the sexual sphere, their hormones are ruled by impulse.

I don't buy it. I have my own fantasy about *Gerald's Game*. In my fantasy, I buy the screen rights to the novel, and like every other director, I turn the plot completely upside down to suit my own taste.

In my story, Jessie and Gerald both have sexual desires they have only recently revealed to each other. They finally have their first open conflict over who's going to be on top. Gerald still gets kneed in the balls, which ends his life. But my Jessie, unlike King's, actually grieves over his death, and she ponders the particular chemistry that drew them together when they were young lovers. While she's thinking up clever ways to escape and reach a glass of water, Jessie runs through her family memories, sparing neither the shame of her night alone with her dad nor the love she still felt for him years later. In my version, she tells her mom and her sister what happened, and the two give contradictory, but always intimate responses. Jessie contemplates a host of sexual memories that have made her the persevering woman she is today.

When Jessie finally escapes, bloody and half-conscious, losing control of her car as she tries to drive for help, I won't have her get rescued by the One Nice Guy in the entire novel. Maybe a woman—a real woman instead of a voice—helps her out. Maybe the dog helps her out.

In the epilogue, as in King's original, I'll have her build her first new relationship with a man. It won't be a lawyer this time, and they're going to follow strict rules of consensuality. When Jessie and—let's call him Chuck—tie each other up, this time they've negotiated a safe word, a word or phrase that brings lovers out of the fantasy and back to the negotiation table. Chuck handcuffs Jessie to the brass posters. She calls out a nasty, intimate name and embraces him with her legs, pulling him closer. He's ready to enter her, she strains against the bed, lifting her hips to pull him in—when all of a sudden there's a low growl, a sickening moan from under the bed.

Chuck pulls the bedspread away from the floor, and Jessie gasps. It's Stephen King, shaking and shuddering, unable to comprehend a shift in the erotic landscape. Jessie can't go on with this monster in the room, and Chuck's hard-on has disappeared. They both scream at King; they are furious, impatient, but determined. "Dammit, Stephen!" they yell together, enunciating their safe words simultaneously, "GROW UP!"

Fermata-cize me!

IT'S VERY LIKELY you've heard of *The Fermata*, the novel by Nicholson Baker. Heralded as "literary smut" by *Publisher's Weekly*, it's a story about a temp worker who has the supernatural ability to stop time on a whim. His favorite pastime while "in The Fold" is to undress and caress appealing women who wander onto his scene. Baker's ero-hero, named Arno, is a Walter Mitty-type personality who smooths back every dress he lifts up, making sure that no woman ever realizes that he's parted her lips, or felt the weight of her breasts in his hands, or inhaled her perfume at close range. He passes the white glove test; he never gets caught.

As a book, *The Fermata* is a good yarn. It has all the necessary ingredients, depending on your inclination, to either arouse you to orgasm or to write a rip-snorting letter to your local paper protesting what an utter piece of filth Nick Baker is. It's fun to read the juicy bits out loud to your lover, and it's even more amusing to read out loud what all the scribes in New York and London have to say about this dastardly pornography from a writer they had thought was such a fine young man. "Good-bye, Nicholson Baker," concluded Victoria Glendinning of the *London Daily Telegraph*, "Good-bye forever."

But forget about the book. By far the most interesting part of *The Fermata* is the parlor game it leaves in your lap. If you had the ability to stop time, what would you do? And even if you erased any trace of your actions, would they still leave a residue? Or is it true that what we don't know can't hurt us? If I'm stripped, fondled, tongued, penetrated, or even spit on by fifty fantasizers a day, does it make any difference if I'm never aware of it?

The last card to be played is whether men, rather than women, have gender-direct tendencies to be psychic peeping toms, constantly undressing the world and having their way with it.

My own *Fermata* parlor game began when I heard the story of a journalist who was so disgusted with *The Fermata's* premise that she set about asking six of her female friends the first thing they would do with themselves if they could stop time.

She triumphantly reported that, in each case, the woman had responded that she would "lie down and take a nap."

Now I assume her friends are all working mothers, but that detail is only the tip of the iceberg. I, too, would love to take a three-hour snooze, but after that bit of refreshment, you'd better believe I'd get into some mischief. I'm nosy, easily titillated, and my imagination has plenty of room for cheap thrills and profound revelations.

I wasn't always this uninhibited about my sexual daydreams. I remember when I was a teenager thinking what a dum-dum I was: while my girlfriends would snicker about what was in some guy's basket, I would still be considering the color of his eyes. Remember the *Sticky Fingers* album that Warhol did for the Rolling Stones? I must have had that album for eight years before I noticed the bulge in the jeans. It was as if my ability to see or notice things below the waist was impaired by a lead shield.

As I became sexually experienced, I realized that I definitely had my preferences when it came to the shape and look of a man's penis, but I still didn't automatically check out crotches unless someone else pointed them out first.

But this is only half the story. Reading *The Fermata* made me realize that I had been undressing women with my eyes for as long as I could remember. It's largely an unconscious behavior; but whenever I'm bored on a plane, in the doctor's office, or at a restaurant, I will often start wondering what the nipples of the woman across from me look like. Or I will fixate on the place where her thighs meet.

My speculation is certainly erotic, but it also goes through all my other feminine lenses, some sexy, some not. My thoughts easily move from cruising, to comparisons with my own body, to feminist fashion outrage, and back again to sordid peeping, all in one *Fermata*-sized minute:

> *Her breasts are so soft and full...I wonder what bra size she wears, bigger than mine?...Where does she buy lacy bras like that, anyway?...All the pretty lingerie only comes in small sizes...anorexic asshole fashion designers...I can just see her in Macy's dressing rooms; her curtain wouldn't close properly and the air conditioning would be on so high that everyone's nipples become stiff...*

Whatever happened to appreciating the art of seeing from a female point of view? Critic Lynn Darling said, in *Esquire's* review of *The Fermata*, that Baker "puts women right where women have always thought men wanted them to be; passive, unaware and not in control of what is happening to them."

Yes, when *YOU*—man, woman, or child—fantasize, the whole world is at your disposal, "passive" and unaware. Whether you're staring at a work of art or the person three seats ahead of you on the bus, only you, the viewer, create the story, the possibilities, the unveiling. To think that men can *look* and *imagine* while women are *blind*, with minds of clay, is preposterous.

Of course, if you insist on walking up to such people on the bus and informing them that they are your love slaves, you are going to be in for a nasty surprise: *reality*. Luckily, most people over the age of two have learned that "let's pretend" is different from genuine cause and effect.

Some people would argue that there is a cumulative effect of voyeurism, a critical mass of objectification that subjugates one class of people under another.

But if the male gaze is what subjugates women, how does that explain homosexual attractions and consequences? A gay man will "objectify" other men he finds attractive; and he will also treat men as his peers, professionally and socially. This very same man may condescend to women and their abilities, never favoring them with a single sexual glance.

Women obviously get fed up with being treated like sex objects all the time, but the pertinent phrase in this complaint is "all the time." There *is* a time and a place for looking at someone with only one thing on your mind. Sometimes we look discreetly, sometimes overtly. If we didn't acknowledge those overt signals, we wouldn't have a species. Men and women thrive on sexual signals, whatever direction they're moving in. To be recognized sexually not only ensures our future, it is an experience that makes us feel alive, however painful or euphoric that may be.

The female sexual gaze has traditionally been ignored—or even worse, punished. There is not a woman alive who hasn't daydreamed about other people's bodies, desires, or possibilities. My preference for looking at tits and biceps, another person's preference for baskets and buns, and still another's exclusive attention to the arches of feet, are entirely unique and not regulated by gender—except insofar as women have a lot more difficulty admitting their erotic interests.

The *only* sexism attached to voyeurism—and this is what is so cruel—is that women have been raised to keep their eyes on the floor! Deference breeds resentment and envy, no doubt about it. Those who cast their eyes downward experience the spectacle of always being looked at and achieving whatever status, high or low, it affords them.

It is the moment when women return the look—and even the stare—that the tables are leveled. *The Fermata* reaches its conclusion exactly this way. Arno finally meets a woman who takes the power of The Fold into her own hands. What good fortune he has encountered. Good-bye, male prerogative, good-bye sleepy deer caught in the headlights—Good-bye forever.

**II.
READING
SEX**

She Knows What She Likes: Dr. Ruth's Illustrated History of Eroticism in Classical Art

OH, THOSE CRAZY Greeks—from the looks of that ancient pottery, they never had a boring moment in bed! And what about that ol' sculptor Rodin? Did he know how to objectify women or what?

Pick your favorite era, pick your favorite artist, give them to pop sex educator Dr. Ruth Westheimer, and watch her trip down art history lane in *The Art of Arousal*, an illustrated coffee-table history of eroticism in classical art. When you get tired of watching her trip, you can stand back for the incredible leaps of faith required to take seriously any of her observations on eroticism or history.

There are two topics that everyone is supposed to know something about but in fact knows next to nothing about—art and sex. Art history is a sorely missed subject in American schools, and Dr. Ruth admits, "When I first started working on this book, I didn't know anything about art." Sex education is even rarer. Nearly everyone gets the sperm-and-egg lecture, but the rest is usually learned on one's own. No other subject is studied in such isolation and secrecy. We are, indeed, a nation of erotic illiterates.

To write on eroticism in classical art demands a certain delicacy and integrity on the part of an author, because it is so easy to take advantage of widespread public ignorance and embarrassment about sexuality. However, in *The Art of Arousal*, Dr. Ruth has no more shame about exposing her unfortunate prejudices than the nudes in the pictures have about shedding their clothes.

The shockers come, not when the author delves into the secrets of human sexuality, but when she does a quick mind-read of the artists and models. Remarking on Rembrandt's portrait, *The Bridal Couple*, she notes that the groom appears to be "an unadventurous lover," and the bride "may never experience orgasm." Similarly, when she critiques a Marisol watercolor depicting several feminine hands reaching out to touch a lover, Dr. Ruth exclaims, "The very long fingernails, especially in the vicinity of a sensitive, erect nipple, are a little worrisome—I don't want anyone to get hurt!"

Some may protest that these remarks are just examples of Dr. Ruth's celebrated sense of humor, which she brings to every discussion of sexual topics. Her idiosyncrasies and her stubborn insistence that people follow particular practices in order to achieve successful sexual lives often evoke the hilarity that has made Dr. Ruth a star on radio and television. If humor is indeed intended in *The Art of Arousal*, we can only wait for other nutty celebrities to do their versions of art history. Just imagine Joe Bob Briggs counting the bare breasts and dead bodies in Jacques-Louis David's *Slaughter of the Innocents*. Or what about Rush Limbaugh doing a critique of the *Mona Lisa* as the smug predecessor of Anita Hill?

However, many of Dr. Ruth's little jokes are less than jovial. Nearly all of her cute comments reflect the most banal retrofeminist posturing; this is manifested in quick blurbs describing male sexuality as an evil empire, denouncing the encroaching pornographic menace, and proclaiming ignorant AIDS alarmism. (After repeated warnings that sex with more than one person is a de facto method of AIDS infection, she goes so far as to counsel, "A dream that includes safer sex is certainly the kind of erotic fantasy best suited to our age.")

Retrofeminism asserts the importance of female orgasm and sexual independence but asserts at the same time that men are sexually distant and dangerous, whereas women are romantic patsies who can only be coaxed by a careful menu of foreplay.

Dr. Ruth's subject—the history of erotic art—deserves to be treated as something other than a male conspiracy. Sex and nudity have been controversial and suppressed in every sort of culture; this history is not a list of anecdotal coincidences, as *The Art of Arousal* seems to imply. The author could easily make the case that erotica has consistently been persecuted in the name of religion and authoritarian obedience. But Dr. Ruth is no pioneer when it comes to erotic politics.

Take her remarks about Auguste Rodin, whom she deconstructs in a manner befitting a Women Against Pornography slide show. The Rodin drawing reproduced in *The Art of Arousal* depicts a woman masturbating while lying on her back, looking into the viewer's eyes. Dr. Ruth projects that "Rodin's model has probably assumed a masturbatory pose but is not actually masturbating." She "looks toward the artist, which seems to have more to do with his fancy (and ego) than hers."

Here's an alternative analysis: Rodin's model is, in fact, a sensual exhibitionist. To be seen and appreciated by her beloved heightens her arousal, and at the very moment Rodin drops his pencil, she reaches orgasm in front of him.

Dr. Ruth's imagination does not stretch this far. She concludes her analysis of Rodin's drawing (along with a similar one by Egon Schiele) by saying, "While it would be easy to dismiss this work as pornography for men—and debasing toward women—these pictures can also be seen as an increasing awareness of women's sexual self-sufficiency."

What on earth makes it so "easy" to dismiss a portrait of a sexually aroused woman as nothing but a vehicle for male selfishness? What is so intrinsically "debasing" about the view between a woman's legs, which the French painter Gustave Courbet very aptly titled *The Origin of the World?*

Rodin's model, who caresses herself so deliberately for this draw- ing, is not demonstrating an "increasing awareness" of anything but her own impending climax.

No female artist who explicitly paints the male or female figure is included in *The Art of Arousal.* This omission dovetails with the sexist assumption that women are incapable of dealing with sex below the waist. How can we have a book published in 1993 that reflects nothing of the powerful renaissance in woman-created erotica?

As a sex education text, *The Art of Arousal* is far from progressive. There is too much in it that suggests that men and women can never communicate with each other about sex, because of men's supposed callousness and women's supposed reluctance. Dr. Ruth makes her most wretched generalization when she insists that "unlike most men, women often desire close contact after orgasm." Such a cruel cliché, that women are not orgasm-oriented and that men don't have a moment to spare for anything else! Dr. Ruth may beg men to behave differently, but her constant pleas and instructions reveal her cynicism.

To say that men and women are different is not saying anything new. What is revelatory about erotica is that it informs us how much passion, sensuality, and responsiveness men and women have in common. Art from all the ages reveals that men and women are equally lusty and tender, both the seducer and the seduced, the corrupt and the innocent. Orgasm is the human response to an erotic imagination, not step-by-step instructions or a politically correct agenda. If we end up talking according to Dr. Ruth's guide to what is good sex, we will inevitably fall silent once again.

III. Sex Lives of the Rich and Famous

I HAVE NEVER had fantastic sex with a groupie. Mind you, I haven't had the opportunities of someone like Mick Jagger, but I have been greeted at the airport by shiny-faced apostles who let me know in the first five minutes that they would do *anything*, anything at all for me. "Anything" usually means they have a list of what they'd like me to do to them, to their bodies, their souls, their memories.

It's the flattery that gets to me. I'm the sort of person to whom you could say, "Oh Susie, you have such pretty hair," and I'd think about it all day. If you lay it on thick enough, I'm likely to feel indebted to you, and that's when the trouble starts.

I know for a fact that I am not as good in the sack as my writing would lead you to believe. Or maybe I am occasionally, but how can I live up to my literary highlights in every motel room on a whistle-stop tour? My performance anxiety with strangers who are attracted to my reputation is so intense that I should just wear a tee-shirt that advertises, "Bad in Bed." My suitors tell me that they are worried that I will write about them in my next story. If only they understood that the real problem is that there might not be anything to write about!

The one thing I don't understand about big-time sex stars is why they NEVER actually talk about their own sexuality. For example, Dolly Parton is known for her huge bosom, but why doesn't she ever talk about whether her breasts are erotic to her? We never hear how sex symbols really feel about sex. When I tell would-be groupies that I am NOT a multi-orgasmic ejaculating Cuisinart, it doesn't make much of a dent, but it reminds them that I am vulnerable, too.

On another plane are the antisex sex stars, the right-wing pundits who make big money and reputations talking about smut all day long. Because they're condemning erotic freedom, we're not supposed to categorize them as sex symbols. But they are! Andrea Dworkin is a sex symbol, so is Jesse Helms. I frankly don't think they have any business talking about other people's preferences if they can't uncloak their own. They get pissed when my crowd says to them, "All you need is a good fuck," as if it weren't a serious suggestion. If right-wing feminists and Christians are having profound and intimate sexual experiences, I want to know. It would be the only thing that would make me listen to them.

The following essays are all based on interviews, gossip, and daydreams about famous people. Dan Quayle ("Dan Quayle's Dick"), of course, is a great beauty and sex symbol who uses his sexual appeal to condemn its consequences. "The Pussy Shot" is an interview with Andrew Blake, a filmmaker whose x-rated success has been attained by fetishizing the trappings of wealth and luxury. Camille Paglia ("Camille Anonymous") is the first American intellectual sexual powerhouse since Emma Goldman, although Emma was a good deal more candid. Angela Barnett ("Lullaby for Angela"), David Bowie's ex-spouse, and my ax-hero Jimi Hendrix ("Having Been Experienced") are both legends of the rock 'n' roll elite, one of the few arenas in the world where it's cool to be sexual, although the costs are big for groupies, wives, handmaidens, and queers.

And if you'll excuse me now, I have to go comb my hair.

Dan Quayle's Dick

I AM A predecessor to Murphy Brown, a single mother before the 1992 election year. When the Family Values camp set up then-Vice President Dan Quayle as its leading spokesperson, I found myself being ideologically pounded almost daily by a man who used single moms and their kids as his punching bag.

I trembled through a series of assassination compulsions as Quayle campaigned from one urban junior high school to the next, insulting eighth graders about their families and fortunes. In two years, after these kids complete puberty, they'll properly knock his lights out for saying such crap to their faces.

Finally, still on the campaign trail, there was the famous spelling bee incident, a humiliation to Quayle's I.Q., but unfortunately not a blow to his moral agenda. I couldn't enjoy his potataux-pas as much as I wanted to. I have inexplicably had consecutive relationships with lovers who are smart as whips but can't spell worth a damn. It's like dyslexia; it's not a matter of intelligence or education at all. Quayle's only real idiocy was to imagine that he should be hanging around a spelling bee in the first place. My other lovers would have had more sense. Our V.P. was impulsive; he forgot who he is and where he belongs.

Once again, Dan spoke out in public without caution on *Larry King Live*. He said that if his daughter were to find herself with child, he would support her, no matter what her decision—whether to keep or abort her pregnancy. He said it twice, and it was the look on his face the first time that made me realize he loved his eldest daughter more than life, that he would do anything for her, and that he could not bear to cause her any pain.

It is a classic father's romance with his little girl. It made me remember when I was a teenager tackling politics with my dad. I belonged to a high school study group that was reading *The Autobi-*

ography of Malcolm X, and I was totally captivated with Malcolm's "by any means necessary" philosophy of self-defense. I decided to battle with my father over his long-standing pacifism.

"What if," I pointed my finger at him like a bayonet, "someone came at you with a gun and your only way to defend yourself was to shoot back?"

He was unshakable. "I would not kill another man," he said. It was like arguing with the Ten Commandments.

I gave up and pouted. "What if someone tried to kill *me*, what would you do then?"

I didn't expect what happened next or I never would have provoked it on purpose. He got that same look that Dan had on TV, his eyes looked a hundred years old, and I was afraid he was going to cry. Then he said, "If it were you, I'd probably do anything to save you." I didn't make him spell it out.

So there was Quayle, cracked and spilt like a yolk, on cable television. The next day, the rest of the Greek drama went into action. Marilyn Quayle rushed right up to the media microphones and told everyone to read her lips. Mrs. Q was furious. If her daughter was pregnant, the girl would "carry the child to term." No ifs, ands, or buts.

Marilyn must have carried *her* pregnancies to term, and raised small children, during times that were not altogether to her liking. She resented it and, like every repressed mother, she was determined to pass on her suffering to her daughters—particularly her eldest daughter, who brought a light to her husband's eyes that he may have stopped sharing with his wife a while back. I feared the romantic love between the Quayles was past. The whole picture made me very sad.

Which brings me to our meeting. I mean, there was absolutely no reason why Danny and I should have had the occasion to meet, let alone exchange bodily fluids with each other....

It happened three nights after his crack-up on the Larry King show.

I was in Washington, D.C., for an anarchist queer conference, with lots of little genderfuck numbers running around—hackers, old yippies. Everyone was crashing at a circle of ancient Victorians near Rock Creek Park.

That's where I had to take Dan. Obviously, one can't run the risk of registering at a motel with him. Just slipping away from the Secret Service is insane enough for a man like him. That's how bad he wanted it.

So let me tell you about *it*, instead of the particulars of how we met.

First of all, Danny says the only important detail about finding me is that he can smell my pussy, "like Girl Scout cookies are supposed to smell," all the way across the park ravine.

You see, Marilyn does not let Danny go down on her. Like maybe she allowed him three times when they were first together, and then it came to a complete halt. Of course, he is just cunt-mad. He buries his head in my fur and simply will not come out—my orgasm is just one curve in the coaster to him. He sucks the cum out of me, licking me like a bowl of chocolate, holding my clit hostage. The only way I can bring him up to eye level is to beg him to fuck me.

And, Geez Louise, his cock is such heaven. I mean, what are the qualifications for a great fuck? Spelling ain't one of 'em. Neither is any kind of brains, let alone progressive politics. Like so many other cruelly teased bimbos, Danny is, bottom line, a very physical and sensual animal who is at his happiest driving balls into holes. The man is an athlete, an Olympian.

For one, he just won't come until I do, long after I do, and then he only pauses to cradle me for a moment and ask if I'm not too sore to carry on. And thanks to a sixteen-ounce bottle of lubricant, I am not in a wheelchair as we speak. His cock is not the biggest dick in America, but it is definitely something to show off.

Of course he's cut, and his erections fly straight up, not curving or bowing. The head looks like a polished marble doorknob—only, it feels, of course, like purple velvet. In fact, his hard-on turns more rosy violet the longer he moves in and out of me. His cock is so pretty that I apologize to him that I am not adept enough to take it all down my throat—I've never been great at that—but he just looks at me like I am crazy and whispers, "Just lick me, baby."

He loves me to tongue the underside of his dick, from the bottom where his balls sit cuddled in anticipation, lapping right up to the cleft in his cockhead. When I suck him this way, he starts whimpering and, needless to say—no, I'll say it again—he crawls inside my pussy once more with his mouth as hungry as a girl's.

Danny sweats like a quarterhorse. His hair, the hair we've all thought of as cemented in Aqua Net, is actually thick and fine and even gets curly when he's down deep between my thighs.

Positions, you ask? My candidate-hero is more than a little romantic. He loves to do it to me like we're making babies, face to face, holding my legs above his shoulders, teasing me with his dick, barely parting my pussy lips—until I grab his arms with all my strength—and try to lift my hips high enough to catch him all the way into my womb.

If being fucked senseless is what I want, he is only too happy to turn me over, never pulling out, just sitting me on my haunches, and stretch my arms out to hold onto the bedrails, because I know what's coming; and he rides me, he rides me holding my hair like a boy clutching a mane, biting my back, and finally, losing his perfect rhythm, talking crazy, gasping, "Do you want me to come inside you, baby?" (Christ, Danny, just keep the condom on, you fool), he takes my hips in his hands like he'd die holding onto me that way and drives me into the ground.

And then I woke up. The bedsheets were soaking wet. I grabbed my Magic Wand, set it on "full term," and finished myself off.

C'mon, I don't want him anywhere near the White House. But wet dreams like this don't visit that often. I only want Dan Quayle sweat-soaked, the cum drained out of him, chained to my bed, just a heartbeat away if I need him.

III. SEX
LIVES OF
THE RICH
AND
FAMOUS

Lullaby for Angela

I never will marry
I'll be no man's wife
I expect to stay single
All the days of my life

WHEN I WAS in fifth grade, one of the most popular pastimes for little girls on the playground was to pose the question: "Which Beatle do you want to marry?" I was so focused on the right answer, as if John, Paul, George, and Ringo were the ultimate multiple choice, that I didn't pay much attention to the rest of the question— *"do you want to marry?"*

I was sexually aroused by listening to the Beatles—my girlfriends and I would play our 45s as loud as we could. We would scream and jump on our beds and tickle each other until we begged for mercy or peed in our pants. Another typical day in prepubescent sexuality.

However, there were other girls, my peers, who had more mature and elaborate plans. These girls planned where they and Ringo would wed, what kind of meals they'd cook for George, how many babies they'd have with Paul, the social asset they'd be to John. These girls took wifeliness as an avocation; their ambitions, not their orgasms, were invested in groupiehood. These girls were very much like Mary Angela Barnett, a.k.a. Mrs. David Bowie.

I met Angela Bowie on her recent tour to promote *Backstage Passes*, her rock 'n' roll memoir that reveals all the "sordid" details of her marriage to the King of Glitter Rock, as well as their acrimonious divorce. Part of her agreement with David was a seven-year gag order that prevented her from publicly discussing her life with him. Angela fell in love with another man, had a daughter, and tried to promote herself artistically without David's coattails to aid her. She had little luck.

"I spent years writing four book proposals that went nowhere," she recalls. "Finally I told my agent to find out what the book publishers wanted, and then call me. I knew exactly when the gag order would end."

What the publishers wanted is indicated in the very first sentence of *Backstage Passes*: "I remember exactly when and where David Bowie and I first slept together."

The book tells us about David's penis, its length, his pet name for it, the strange rash he gets from intercourse. The details are often explicit, but rarely intimate. Although Angie "tells all," her book reveals little of her inner life, sexual or otherwise.

Her marriage seems to begin more as a business affair than a romance. David wanted to be a star, and Angie wanted to *make* him one. They made a pact: she would devote herself to his career, and when he got on top, he'd do the same for her.

Well, you'll never guess what happened: her efforts were not reciprocated. Her theatrical aspirations were unrealized. She doesn't say so in the book, but I could easily see the faces of all the producers who took one look at her bio, her background, her audition, and wondered what the prospects were of exploiting David Bowie's wife.

I have never had an interview with a "wife" before, and I doubt I will have one with a "husband" in such circumstances. When I remember female rock stars who've been exposed by their ex's, I think of Janis Joplin, Tina Turner, Cher. They are all described as hurt little girls looking for love, unprepared to handle their talent, and indebted to men who made them work their asses off.

David Bowie is not described by Angie or anyone else as a hurt little boy. He needed mothering, of course, but not in the sentimental sense. He needed someone to plan ahead, fend off, clean up the mess, make a nice home, bear him an heir. He was ready to exploit his talent, and as Angie puts it, "David always had the drive to get what he needed." The only female star to whom this characteristic is ascribed is Madonna, whose femininity suffers because she is considered too ambitious, and therefore too much like a man.

No one will accuse Angela Bowie of losing her femininity by publishing a kiss-and-tell book. Hers is a classic female persona, the power behind the throne who is cast off and waits for her revenge, preferably eaten cold. Her story is as simple as this: "I gave my man everything, and he betrayed me."

I had only one real question for Angela Bowie, perhaps the most difficult question: "What is it like for your identity to be defined by your relationship to a man?" I never see this question asked in *Vanity Fair*. I never hear anyone ask Princess Di, or Ivana, or Jerry Hall, "What does it do to you to be valued for your relationship to another, to the man who impregnated you, whose status you wear on your finger—a man who leaves you with nothing but abandonment?" The magazines never ask these questions. Instead they make a fuss over these women's beauty, education, and background, as if these are qualities that catapulted them to fame. (Angela told me five times in our interview that she had been reared at the very best Swiss schools, "to be the biggest tycoon I could be." Later I asked myself, are the female graduates of Montreaux running the world? No, but they are married to men who are.)

How would Angela answer my unavoidably cruel question? At best, I hoped she would describe a sense of dignity, an explanation for what it means to really help someone who has a rare gift. Perhaps bringing that gift to acclaim without necessarily seeing your own name in lights provides a quiet, sane satisfaction that has not been truly appreciated.

I had imagined she might tell me a "recovery" story, a drama of codependency and liberation, a struggling inner child, a therapist who asked all the right questions.

I knew from reading *Backstage Passes* what Angela was *not* going to do. She was not going to offer a fiery analysis of how women are men's chattel, with herself as just one more drop in the bucket of oppression. But I wondered if she had considered that view for even a moment.

Her answer was none of the above. "I know you're sincere," she began. "But your questions are irrelevant. I'm a great marketer. The product was David Bowie.

"I think kissing and telling is just fine. The gossip was all over the tabloids, and if I'm smart enough to put together my story in a book, more power to me. I've got stuff to do! Deadlines, a daughter to raise. I'm not worried about whether people trust me. I'm not running for president. These concerns are asinine, juvenile. I'm interested in effectiveness. I'm a colonel's daughter, you know, and there is a job to be done."

I didn't know how to reply. I thought I had asked the most relevant question possible for a woman in her position, and she had swatted it like a fly.

She relented slightly: "Look, I had ulcers when I was nineteen, trying to make David the very best. Ulcers are not for me.

"After my *job* with David was over, I had to pay dues, do everything from the beginning...I would go to auditions where I was treated like a bimbo and I would lose my temper. It infuriated me, I'm too much of a snob, and I didn't get any jobs acting that way. But I didn't have any choice.

"The worst thing is that I went directly from promoting David Bowie to promoting my next love, Andrew Bogdan Lipka, the father of my daughter, which is exactly what I promised myself not to do. It was easy, like falling off a log for me."

"So why haven't you fallen off the log again?" I asked.

She gave me an abbreviated story. "Andrew started drinking terribly and finally got himself shot. But he lived, and when he was on the operating table and I was standing there, I thought, 'This is my last chance, this is my last chance to do something for myself, and if I fall, I'll be picking myself up, not someone else.' "

"Is that how we change?" I wondered, "through a single cataclysmic event?" I find that such events work like diets, and you put all the weight back on without a serious overhaul. I have looked at my own past in this regard, and I decided to take another peek at Angela's.

I opened her book to the photo section. There is only one photograph of Mary Angela as a child, and it is quite extraordinary. She has pure blond hair, curled and combed down her back; a lace, pearl, and taffeta dress, white anklets, and white patent leather shoes, legs crossed, hands posed in her lap. She is smiling, but not too much, no teeth, just one corner of her mouth turned up. Am I a good girl? Am I the colonel's daughter? Yes. Yes. Yes.

This portrait is across the page from a chapter entitled, "Bisexual Boogie."

"How come there wasn't a section in your book where you came out to your parents?" I asked. "You know, where they flipped out about your rock 'n' roll and genderbending life." She laughs. "It's not there," she looks straight at me. "Because it didn't happen."

I don't believe her. She is contradicting her book and the stories she's told me. One minute she rebukes my lesbian inquiries, snorting, "I never put my head between anybody's anything." Later, she recalls seducing an extra on the set of *The Man Who Fell To Earth*. "She got herself seriously satisfied," Angie smiles. "If I'm drunk enough, I can be butch enough." My eyes widen; it's the first time she has used gay vernacular with me. I notice she has uncrossed her legs, and her navy blue skirt is hitched up over her knees. She has never had her portrait taken this way.

I press her again about the husband-free identity. "I am famous," she exclaims, emphasizing the *I*, "because I was expelled from the Connecticut College for Women for having a lesbian affair." True enough, I can imagine the commotion she caused in 1960-something. The last time Angela Barnett was recognized on her own was as a disgraced and stigmatized undergraduate. She says she has never fallen in love with a woman again.

I went to get my car serviced after the interview and boasted to my mechanic that I had just had tea with Angela Bowie.

"She didn't really find Mick in bed with David, did she?" he begs. I can see his worst fears are coming unglued over the Rolling Stones half of that equation.

"Oh Jake, that's old news already," I say. "Everyone knows those guys are bisexual."

What a revelation. It is not even who Angela *fucked* that made her famous, it's who she observed fucking, who she watched from the end of the bed.

She has written her memoir from the end of a bed and from a terrible distance. Her presence is a guarded shadow, a white pearl of denial. She is a watchful daughter with a half smile who says, without blinking, it's not here, it's not there, because it never really happened.

Camille Anonymous

GLORIA STEINEM CAN relax. Tell Naomi Wolf there's no reason to feel singled out. Feminists and sensitive intellectuals around the world can just let their hair down because I, too, have received my very own hate mail from Camille Paglia. I won't hide the fact that Camille has dressed me down in two blistering pages of her own handwriting.

"Why *you?*" you máy ask, and so did I. I was even flattered at first, because I couldn't imagine why she had spent her precious time reducing me to a loathsome little worm. But now I realize I am common. My plight is banal. So many people have received hate mail from Paglia that we are now ready for our own recovery group. Our first step: admit we are powerless over Camille.

I'm sure I'll be attending C.A. meetings with her ex-car mechanics, her ex-hairdressers, her ex-lovers, and of course her chain of intellectual nemeses.

I'll get up from my little wooden folding chair and tell the naked truth: I couldn't stop reading Camille—not only her books, which can only be completed on drugs, but her incredible media blasts, her screamingly funny retorts to everything from Monday night football to kiddie porn.

My friends tried to warn me; they said, "Camille Paglia is not a laugh. She is not a wit. *She is a tool of the right wing.*"

"Hey, you are dead wrong," I told them. "Camille is not a tool—she is a *weather* phenomenon." And if you think Pat Buchanan calls up Hurricane Camille for strategy sessions, you've got another thing coming. This is the woman who championed man/boy love on Philadelphia daytime television.

Monkey wrench, maybe; tool, *never.*

When I first met Camille, she was an unknown face. She came to a reading of my book *Susie Sexpert's Lesbian Sex World,* a couple of months after she released her own *Sexual Personae.* She popped up during my lecture like a jack-in-the-box on methedrine, saying she was my "only friend in academia" and laying into the fragile institution of liberal humanities like she was punching the Pillsbury doughboy right in the kazoo.

Her ferociousness took me aback. Of course I've had my own battles with a certain *Prime of Miss Jean Brodie* atmosphere that turns women's studies undergraduates into soldiers against pornography. But I've also made allies in the ivory tower who are sexually adventurous and thoughtful. I wondered how Camille could imagine she was the only one. I interviewed Camille almost a year later, in a two-hour phone call. I was delighted to learn that she was willing to discuss how her theories about sex intersected with her own sex life.

Sometimes she'd hold up a fig leaf of privacy to my more outrageous questions, but I thought it was a great improvement over the time I asked Susan Sontag at a lecture what she thought of lesbian pornography, and she turned her head away like someone had taken a dump on the carpet.

Camille, on the other hand, was candid about her life and childhood, and how they influenced her ideas. She saw herself as unique at nine years old, as she does today.

She also admitted to me that she exaggerates to make a point; she thinks of it as guerrilla word-fare. I understood that immediately. Camille's critics imagine that she would pass by a woman getting raped on the street and only sneer, "She asked for it." Nothing could be further from the truth. Paglia is the type who would fight a man twice her size if he was even condescending to a woman, let alone violating her. Right makes might in Camille's battles for justice, and no one can outdo her righteous authority.

But you know, everyone is touchy about something, and Camille finally pushed my button. She opened an essay in *Playboy* with a boast I could not tolerate: "I am a pornographer," she wrote.

"You are *not!*" I screamed in my bed, where I ordinarily love to feast on Camille clippings. My vibrator clattered to the floor. "What do you know about being persecuted for sex?" I sneered at her picture in which, of course, she was fully clothed.

Whatever criticism gets leveled at Camille, she's not going to jail for dissing Susan Faludi. Furthermore, nobody will call her a slut or a bimbo as long as she keeps her clothes on, which is this country's criterion for respecting women. She is an academic, not an activist or a "purveyor of obscene material," and so her risks are different. I resented her putting on the faux cloak of porn. Finally, I was offended!

Many Camille-aholics say this is the first step toward recovery, but in my case it only upped the ante. The fact is I'm a tolerant person by nature, and I wasn't about to disown my affection for her overnight. Underneath it all, I really wanted to run wild with Camille, take in a few live sex shows, stay up all night. So when it was announced she was coming to San Francisco to lecture at the Herbst Theatre, I faxed her a little note suggesting we paint the town red. Never heard from her.

Meanwhile, I was invited by the Herbst show organizers to interview her on stage. I thought that would be a blast. I wanted to show slides of classical art and contemporary photography to elicit her stream of consciousness reactions. I wanted to tease her and provoke her and seduce her on stage.

Well, things did not turn out that way. I was treated to a platter of obfuscation. Camille never talked to me, but various intermediaries did; they said that Camille was actually doing her act solo, and I could introduce her if I liked. I didn't appreciate the string of middlemen. Why couldn't she talk to me for five minutes? That ticked me off and baffled me as well. Camille was not making her customary direct hit.

After her successful show, reporters were all over, hoping to get an outraged feminist reaction, or at least an outraged something. I pulled a Lloyd Bentsen with some microphone jockey, saying, "Camille, you're no pornographer."

But what a performance artist she was. The two hours had flown right by, and we all would have stayed for more. She appealed to anyone who ever stuck his or her head out a window and screamed, "I'm mad as hell, and I'm not going to take it anymore." She was unabashedly sexual in her intellect and passionate about not caring what anyone thinks—a quality rare in women.

Two months after Paglia's lecture, I was in bed with a bout of pneumonia. An envelope from the University of the Arts in Philadelphia arrived. It was from Camille. It was the meanest thing ever addressed to me in my life.

She was furious that I had not introduced her at the Herbst. How dare I say she had not "paid the price of her beliefs"?

"I have been 'unemployed'," she retorted, "unpublished, kicked out of one job, insulted to my face."

She called me solipsistic, a diva, and naïve. "Wake up to

reality...establishment feminism has destroyed women's education. Don't you see the destructiveness of the date-rape hysteria? I've taken more abuse on that alone than you *ever* have—hostility and defamation from Alaska to Miami...You lost big by your behavior toward me this trip."

I trembled at what my punishment might be, and she delivered it in the inky postscript: "I *had* been speaking positively about your new book—all this is now over. You have shown your true colors."

Yikes! If I hadn't gotten my next cortisone shot in the minutes following her letter's revelations, I might have dropped dead on the spot.

Had I finally reached my bottom, was I willing to say no to the abuse?

Not yet.

I spent the next day writing Camille a very nice letter, saying I wished she had spent just a moment talking to me in person so things hadn't gotten so ugly. I told her that receiving even one boo, hiss, or death threat was more than enough, that I didn't mean to belittle the risks she'd taken with her career. I told her not to believe everything she read in the paper. I wrote, "I am not your enemy."

I hoped that this approach was gallantly turning the other cheek, rather than exhibiting my abject codependency. How could she go from being my *only* friend in academia to my most virulent adversary?

The last straw arrived the day after Christmas, I got another envelope from the University of the Arts—this time, a big folder. Inside was my *unopened* letter, and the following message on letterhead:

"Due to the overwhelming volume of international mail, Professor Paglia cannot accept unsolicited packages, manuscripts or gifts. Nor does she have time to read or review poems, articles, essays, theses, books, videotapes, slides, or art works. Packages are opened by staff and their contents discarded, unless return postage has been enclosed."

My goodness.

I was so inspired I've now made up my own form letter which simply states, "Susie Bright does not accept unsolicited hate mail."

I've laid my confession bare, and you can see how old habits die hard. I've made amends to friends and family. I've come to believe that the Higher Power of Utter Indifference is the only thing that can save me. But damn you, Camille, you great big nut, I just had to write about you one more time.

The Pussy Shot:
An Interview with Andrew Blake

I'M IN A beach side luxury hotel room with a forty-five-year-old man I've never met before, yet whom I've fantasized about for years. I've got several adult videos lying on my king-size bed, ones that I've seen dozens of times before, but never with him.

I ask him shyly to pick out his favorite while I pull the drapes, so the room is as cool and dark as a projection booth. Usually when I'm with a man and we've got any "porn shopping" or choosing to do, the fellow always defers to me. It's like the new chivalry of adult video: ladies' choice. Men are so thrilled that at least some women *want* to watch dirty movies that they're willing to adapt to any subject matter in order to ensure an enjoyable evening.

But back to my own private guest of honor. I believe he's even more nervous than I am, and it was remarkable that he agreed to meet me here at all. I ask if he minds if I start rolling tape now, and he shakes his head. I've waited for this for so long...

My special date to watch blue movies is with Andrew Blake, the erotic-film director who has single-handedly defined the birth of yuppie porn. Remember what *Miami Vice* did to cop shows? This is what Blake's brand of L.A. vice did to the modern porn biz. Blake is the creator of such modern classics as *Night Trips, House of Dreams*, and *Hidden Obsessions*. His million dollar sex films have virtually no script or dialogue but thrive instead on lavish art direction and editing.

Art direction for Blake, who was a painter before he was a pornographer, means using locations that look like dream vacations, bodies that look like they rose off the foam, and styling and design from *Architectural Digest* instead of a porn set. His movies have been enormously successful with both male and female viewers who are aroused by a touch of class, and they've been just as annoying to people who prefer their sex mouthy and raw.

I have to say that I identify with the latter. My first reaction to Blake's films was that they were like a hardcore version of a yuppie lingerie catalog.

"I suppose this is what some *90210* prick thinks women want," I sneered. I'd rather see a woman begging for and screaming her orgasm in a ditch than watch her nonchalantly finger herself in an art deco foyer.

But I was not the only one weighing in my opinions. My sister-in-law called me up one night after celebrating her wedding anniversary at one of those adult motels with cable TV. She had watched *Hidden Obsessions.* "I want to see every film this guy Blake has ever made," she told me. Not long after her confession, I walked in on my lesbian baby-sitter one midnight watching the girl-girl scene from *House of Dreams* in slow-motion. She was drooling!

Aside from such moving personal testimonies, I saw Blake's videos fly out the door at my local women's sex boutique. Clearly I was being a reverse snob—something about Blake's movies was clicking with real couples, real women, not to mention the men who form his traditional audience.

Back at my hotel room, Andrew picks *House of Dreams* to slip in the VCR, apparently concurring with my baby-sitter's preferences. We watch the opening together as a Paulina Porizkova lookalike named Zara White stretches out in a pale bedroom with her lush body as its centerpiece.

"Where do you come up with these luxury mansions with nothing in them?" I ask.

"In Los Angeles," he says, deadpan.

Blake is more relaxed looking at the screen than facing me; his eyes are thinking, expressive. I know this is what he looks like when he looks through a lens, and seeing this professional voyeurism, if you will, makes me more excited than I've ever been in front of his movies.

"Do your movies show what you genuinely think is sexy?" I ask. "Or did you conduct careful research in the advertising world to find out that—"

"No, no, I hate research. I didn't care what the market would tolerate. When I first did these films, there were people who were saying 'Oh, if only he could be dirtier.' But I really wasn't doing them for that group. You know, the *Hustler* set."

Class comparisons are Blake's point of entry, and it makes me squirm. I find it diabolical that standards of sexiness are delineated by such strict ghettos—elite, highbrow erotica versus. those awful white-trash porn addicts across the tracks. Why is a straight-on shot of a woman's vulva considered debauched? Why do the proper tan lines make *all the difference*? Do educated middle-class people really have such different fantasies from high school drop-outs with bad hair? I beg to differ.

I decided to put it to him this way: "What's so erotic about wealth?"

"It's what I like to see," he says, not particularly defensive. "Very beautiful girls in very sexy situations. I'm not approaching it from the point of view of displaying an unbelievably garish house or whatever. But if I'm going to see a beautiful girl, why do I need to see her in a dump? It's like the fashion image—beautiful clothes, beautiful women, beautiful furniture. It's not about wealth, it's about beauty."

The star on screen rubs her cunt, and her mouth trembles open, just slightly. Her pussy lips are small like mine. It's the first thing that begins to pass my wet test, which in turn makes me feel the tension of trying to run a professional interview when I'd just as soon start playing with myself. Our Zara wets her finger in her cunt, and I notice that her pussy is perfectly composed with every hair in place, a fashion detail which allows me to recover my equilibrium.

"How similar are the fantasies you direct from your own sex life?" I ask.

"There are certain situations that are the same," he says. "I guess I've led a very designed life. I live in a very beautiful house, I drive a beautiful car—boy, I'm quoting some songwriter now, aren't I? I like to surround myself with nice things. So this is kind of an outgrowth of that."

Something not so nice is on screen now. It's a couple, all in blue, with fluorescent orange highlights on the girl's accessories. Like her fake nails, for instance, which Blake shakes his head at. "This didn't turn out like I wanted, it's too crass."

We share a few moments questioning *why*—since everyone agrees that fake nails, too-big hair, and plastic tits are a turn-off—does every actress in the business seem destined for all three. It's like this awful curse that can't be broken without a virgin's touch—not likely in this crowd. I hand him the remote so we can fast forward through this scary blue blow job.

Blake freezes the screen just as Zara appears in a leather collar, locked into place by a severe leather femme top.

"Here we have Jeanna Fine, pre-boob job. She was really into this.

And I believe she was a professional dominatrix for a while. I think that this scene is one of the best scenes in the movie...."

Jeanna starts tracing her crop stick around Zara's ass cheeks and circling her cunt hairs.

"This is the part where I wanted Jeanna to stick the magic wand up inside her," I say. "This is very teasy." I can vicariously feel what it's like for her pussy lips to be waiting, anticipating something to go inside.

"Yes," Andrew nods slightly.

This must be the scene my baby-sitter enjoys so much. I pound the mattress a little in impatience. Now the bottom girl is getting fucked, but it's not enough to rock her boat. The New Age music in the background is driving me batty. It seems the history of the porn soundtrack has gone from Montovani rip-offs to Aerobic Disco, and now to something that sounds like a slightly cheaper version of *The Piano* soundtrack. I hate them all, but I can't really bring myself to press "mute" because then I would miss any yummy groaning and gasping.

"Words would help a lot with this kind of scene." I say. "You have no dialogue. I'd appreciate a little blistering S/M discourse. Not a corny one, but a good one!"

Blake's attention is squarely on Jeanna, who starts fucking Zara standing up, with a special dildo headpiece.

"Did this deliver for you?" Andrew asks. It's interesting he's using the past tense, since I'm feeling everything I've ever felt right now.

"Mmmmmmmm, no, not nasty enough. I like the push and pull here, but it's so formal..."

"For me it was an *exotic* visual, I'd never seen a device like this before, and—"

"Yes. It is exotic, and I like that Zara is so precarious on her high heels, but I want that feeling of precariousness enhanced by her being fucked really hard. I want to see that she can hardly take it, see her trembling. *I want to make her come.* In this heterosexual idea of girl-girl sex, it's all foreplay."

Now Blake is interested. "So how do lesbians themselves feel about het-produced lesbian scenes?"

"Well, of course the party line is that all lesbians hate it," I say. "But there's a lot of different opinions. I am personally attracted to butch women, so these lipstick lesbians in straight movies leave me cold. I'm always looking at the lesbian scenes, trying to find the one who's secretly butch—the one who knows how to use her hands.

A masculine or androgynous woman is what makes my clit jump."

"So that androgynous quality is really what is exciting to you?"

"Yes, but do I look androgynous? No, not at all, but I'm attracted to my opposite in—"

"Okay, I got it, that's your personal taste," he nods. "There shouldn't be one politically correct-looking woman, or man, for that matter."

It's interesting he's saying that, since his models are the conventional model type. I want him to really understand the whole nature of what is politically correct in an un-straight world.

"Lesbians find themselves right in the middle of this 'classic beauty' argument," I tell him. "Some dykes find the *Playboy* woman to be their ideal, and others find her to be an ideal but they feel guilty about her. Some dykes don't find the centerfold type ideal, and it has nothing to do with their politics, they just honestly desire a different kind of woman. That is the most unique position to have, because it's hard to separate your feelings from what everybody says you should be feeling."

"Okay," he says. "But in terms of the girl-girl scenes in the films that I do, my motivation is to see these two beautiful works of art together, these two women. I'm not consciously looking to create a fantasy where the man is going to bust in and service them."

I make a face as soon as he says "works of art," but he's not deterred.

"I guess a lot of people think of my movies as being very detached," he continues. "You don't get up close and intimate, people don't get sweaty, they're not as animalistic as some people would like. The actors remain too perfect. I guess that's my prejudice, but I don't particularly like showing bad body angles or cellulite, or—"

"Yeah, but showing cellulite is different from showing somebody being drenched and exhausted…"

I check the screen to realize that the lesbian business is over and now actor Rocco Sifreddi is unsnapping a woman's garter in one swift move.

"I've always been impressed with the lover who can unsnap you like that…In fact, I've never had one."

"Yes. Those are the ones I'm looking for. Who can do it in one take." Blake scans the picture. "Now we have the dual blow job."

Two femme heads, blond and brunette, lick up and down the actor's penis like a syncopated swizzle stick. This might as well be an exercise tape.

"Do you like that?" I ask, since he pointed it out.

"Ah, I thought it worked. Nice composition, they both are into it. Rocco looks in control."

I am aware of Rocco's reputation. "Yeah, women fans love his cock. They think he has a pretty...dick."

We pause to watch Rocco come into one woman's mouth, who daintily lets the semen drop like a pearl to the point of the other girl's high heel, which poses directly below her chin.

"Mmhm," Andrew hums. "This I like very much. The shoe, the face, and the dick."

"Yes, it's your very best shoe facial," I congratulate him. "Do you have admiration for the male actors, somebody you think is really hot?"

"No. Actually, if I could pull all the men out, I would."

"Tell me why!" This is the tenth porn director who's told me this. I wonder if it's universal, four out of five, or what. No wonder most straight porn looks so uninspired.

"I guess I just like looking at women rather than men," he answers.

"But your films don't exclusively focus on women," I press him. "They focus on men *with* women. Isn't that as beautiful as women together or alone?"

"I look at the man as a prop. A piece of furniture."

That makes me laugh and Andrew does too. But he's so careful— "Again, it's just my own gut reaction to these things."

"I know! I want to know more about your guts."

"I would just prefer looking at women. In some of the shots that I do, I'll have the couple together, but I'll avoid showing the man, so the viewer can, or *I* can, 'put my face there.' "

The screen has suddenly turned golden and we've arrived at the last beach scene.

I remember this scene very well and it's a perfect example of what we've been talking about. "Now this is a situation where your prejudice against the boy was obvious," I say. "Here's this blond surfer boy who jumps onto the beach, and I want to objectify his body, enjoy him—and you're completely ignoring him!"

"On the other hand, we have our two beach women."

"Yeah, the two mermaids." Big deal.

Mermaid A starts toying with Mermaid B. I find this scene intensely irritating. "No lesbian would ever fuck somebody like that." I declare. "This is a wash for me."

"You mean, just the position of her hands, or the way she was doing it?"

"The way she's doing it, with one ring finger!" I'm disgusted. "The natural position is to use either your index or middle finger, and most likely, more than one. Or your thumb!" I want to say something else which is complicated. "I can't tell from looking at the movie what these actresses' preferences really are, because some real-live dykes are in this business and put on incredibly phony scenes. But this performance makes me doubt this model's lesbian credibility."

Blake explains his point of view. "See, my feeling was that if she penetrated her completely, then you wouldn't see...."

"Yes, this is the problem, you *can't see*, you can't show the sex feelings *on the inside*, that's very difficult. Some of the hottest real life sex in looks like beached whales on camera."

"Exactly."

"So why don't you show women coming?" This is my gripe to end all gripes. "You love women in front of the camera, but you never show them getting off."

I don't mean to single Blake out, because the entire X-rated business ignores female orgasm. The irony is that the Number One question I get asked by men who come to me for erotic advice is where they can find movies where women climax on-screen. With all the attention to the guy's come shot, the male fan apparently wants to see the female come shot.

Andrew questions me back. "Do you think my stuff doesn't portray that, the woman's arousal, is that what you're saying?"

"Well, very often you tease, tease, tease," I say, "but I don't see the climax. I remember in your *Night Trips* with superstar Tory Welles, where I had the feeling that she was coming, but—"

"Then I cut it away?"

"Yes! I wanted to kill you! This guy was doing Tori from behind, and she was holding onto something, getting very aroused, and all of a sudden you pulled from a close-up to a medium shot. Here I was, dying to see the flush on her chest, her sweat—I wanted to see her mouth when she came! I wanted to see her clit swollen and her pussy contracting. Jesus!"

"That's a good point. I guess I'm guilty of that."

"Well, why are you guilty?"

"Sometimes it just doesn't happen. Not that it couldn't be portrayed as happening—"

"Of course, look at all the other faking that goes on!"

"I'm guilty, I'm guilty."

For some reason I can't stop myself from putting the screws in.

"Don't you like it in real life when your partner comes? Isn't it part of what gets you off?"

"Oh, absolutely."

"Well, why is it, like, not happening in your movies?"

"I guess I build up to it, maybe I don't deliver it all the time, but I try to do my best. What can I say? That's a valid criticism. Okay?"

I might as well get him to sign on the dotted line now. I never thought I'd have the most famous porn director doing a *mea culpa* number with me on the issue of female orgasm. It's my own private *Hite Report* moment.

"So does this mean that in your next movie you're going to make sure that the women come?" I ask.

"Yeah, that would be fine. Yeah."

"Why don't you invite me, and I'll be the orgasm verifier?"

We've got just enough time to be quiet and watch the final scene with Zara listening to a seashell as if her fantasy were contained inside its spiral. Andrew jumps up from his chair to switch off the tube, and I, more slowly, unplug my mike and open the curtains. If I were alone, I'd masturbate now. I can't watch sex for this long—good, bad, or otherwise—without wanting to pull some of it into my own body.

If we were real bohemians, I'd just do it, wouldn't I? But instead, I'm shaking Blake's hand and walking him to the door. Good luck, good-bye, may all your money shots be pussy happy. I pull the curtains dark again and stick in another tape. Somebody's got to finish those girls off.

Having Been Experienced: Jimi Hendrix, and Why the Little Dykes Understand

TEENAGERS FIND REASONS to live and die in popular music. The aging process grinds this passion to a halt, as we simultaneously become more cynical and cautious. But a former teenager never forgets her first, and my first was Jimi Hendrix.

Hendrix is one of the most compelling legends of the '60s. He was a virtuoso musician, a "fuckin' genius" as they say, and he died at the height of our country's discontent, an estrangement he described many times in his lyrics. He deliberately commented on society's rules and wages of war. He was an army veteran who was not a stranger to the term "imperialism." For these reasons, I idolized him, not as a revolutionary guitarist, but as a revolutionary *and* an ax man.

Yet there was something about Jimi's sound, rather than the lyrics or the times he lived in, that made young people, and in particular me, want to be *free*, in that classic sense of no inhibitions, no limits, no authority.

When I talk to men of my generation who revere Hendrix, they usually rap about his technical mastery and mysteries. But the largest mystery to me about Hendrix was not how he achieved his outlandish distortion, but how he made my *world* seem so distorted—why my body responded to his voice, why *"If six turned out to be nine, I don't mind, I don't mind."* I've been playing *Electric Ladyland* for twenty years now, but I didn't examine what Jimi meant to me until I had a very weird flashback in the mid-'80s...

It's hard to keep track of all the military actions the United States has engaged in since Vietnam. Since Nixon, every Pentagon folly is an incident, a "warette," and in that vein, perhaps you recall that in 1986, Reagan bombed Libya.

I remember the day the Libyan air strike was reported because I was at a lesbian strip show that night. It was a Tuesday, the night I co-hosted a women-only strip club. This evening was our usual two hundred-plus crowd of leatherdykes, financial-district escapees, and Midwestern tourists. The strippers were all local girls who worked regularly at the downtown sex clubs.

The kind of erotic dancer who plays to a dyke crowd tends to have a bit more spirit, a real desire to connect to the crowd. But their costumes and acts were rarely different from what they'd perform at a regular porn palace, regardless of their sexual orientation.

They all danced to Top Forty, which at the time was a string of tunes by Janet Jackson, Mötley Crüe, Vanity. It was an '80s crowd with an '80s beat, and the last thing I expected to hear any Tuesday was the electrified rattle of a machine gun.

It was *the* "Machine Gun," Jimi Hendrix's song from *Band of Gypsys* circa 1970. The first riffs erupted on a bare stage, and then a yellow spot came up. Out of the darkness, a stripper named Lupe crawled on her belly upstage, in a combat uniform and a gas mask. She was a death spirit; her body was contorted and furious, and her sexuality was driven by Hendrix's ferocious *rat a tat tat*.

She did her entire set, seventeen minutes, to Hendrix's anthem, and the gas mask was the one thing that never came off.

I don't know what the girls at the cocktail tables were thinking; I don't know if cruising and foreplay came to a halt. Most of the audience was younger than I: I don't think they remembered Walter Cronkite announcing the number of Vietnam casualties every night. Some of these baby dykes may have been born the year that Hendrix played his disintegrated version of "The Star Spangled Banner" at Woodstock, which became the theme song of everyone—including myself—Who Would Rather Be Smashing the State.

Lupe was old for a stripper—almost thirty. When she came off the stage, she was so soaked I didn't know if it was tears dripping off her face or sweat. But when she saw my own tearful face as I hugged her, she began to cry in earnest. "You know why I did it, you know," she said, and when she got a little drier, I asked her how she started listening to Jimi.

We had both listened for umpteen hours to Hendrix's "Machine Gun," which was released during the most political and "black" phase of his career. She and I remembered smoking a lot of pot to this album, mucho peyote, making love to both men and women, and cursing the United States of Ameri*kkk*a. It was a time of *inverted* patriotism, where the very thing that made you hate LBJ, the Pentagon, Tricky Dick, and how-many-kids-he-killed-that-day, was the same thing that made you think that maybe this country had some greatness after all, if only we could get rid of the pigs. At that time I considered corporate greed to be a cancer on the body; I still trusted we were born clean.

I have one unusual clue to my feminine Hendrix fascination, which tied my revolutionary interest in him to my sexual interest. Everyone who has read the postmortem Hendrix biographies has heard tell about Jimi's huge sexual appetite, his big dick, and his black erotic presence in a white milieu.

But in the middle of my lesbian strip show years, I found unexpected pictures and clues in the record of his life. One of Hendrix's closest running buddies had been a woman named Devon—his lover, roommate, pimp, dealer, and advisor. She was often called a "super groupie," linked with Mick Jagger and others. But the most interesting thing I read about her was that she was a bisexual, a hooker who reputedly only loved women but fucked men for money and advantage. That would describe most of the women I met at our lesbian burlesque.

Devon's bisexuality is not commented on very much in the typical Hendrix bio except to say that Jimi "straightened Devon out." I thought that notion was very funny, because my reading of a woman like Devon is that she queered Jimi *in*.

Hendrix wrote a song about his muse, called "Dolly Dagger," which one official biographer claimed was a mocking rhyme about Devon's relationship with Jagger. But this rock journalist obviously didn't know the biggest contribution Black English has made to the queer vernacular: bulldagger. Dolly/Devon was a bulldagger *par excellence*.

> *Been riding broomsticks since she was fifteen*
> *Blowin' out all the other witches on the scene*
> *She got a bullwhip just as long as your life*
> *Her tongue can even scratch the soul out of the devil's wife*
> *Well, I seen her in action at the player's choice*
> *Turning all the love men into doughnut boys*

I wondered if "doughnut boys" meant guys who couldn't wait to get Dolly's cock up their ass. Instead of imagining Hendrix's big dick, I saw his begging asshole in my mind and Dolly taking him with her magic broom dick. After all, men who haven't gotten down on their knees don't say " *'scuse me while I kiss the sky*."

I find it absolutely plausible '90s that Hendrix was a dyke daddy, a fellow traveler, and that the queer femme lacing to his soul was something I could anchor my militant teenage sexuality to. Of course, I am practicing the ultimate Spectator's Choice, making my hero into me, believing that we shared a faith rather than just a good beat we could dance to.

 Hendrix introduced me to the blues, to funk, and to divine cacophony. If I hadn't been fifteen at the time, I would have been unable to hang my political and erotic identity on his hook. But I was lucky.

Sure, I think lots of MTV stars are cute, but I don't see them when I look out my belly button window. I've fantasized fucking many rock 'n' roll legends, but I've never again had the feeling I got with Hendrix that I could fuck the whole wide world.

With Jimi you could love it *and* leave it; the two philosophies were not exclusive. He carved an axis bold as love and left me like he left so many others—spinning in it.

HAVING
BEEN
EXPERI-
ENCED

IV. Sex in America

RECENTLY, A PROMINENT university library called to ask my advice on acquisitions of pornographic films; they had been given a private donation to expand their collection. This university's film department has made quite a name for itself studying pop culture cinema, of which pornography is certainly the largest category. Yet from an academic perspective, porn has been almost impossible to research. I make a habit of looking up "pornography" in the card catalog of any library I happen to visit, and usually the only books listed are calls-to-antiporn-arms by Catharine MacKinnon and Andrea Dworkin, and Linda Lovelace's *Ordeal.* In other words, by checking the library, it's easy to find out why we should ban porn; but you'd be hard pressed to find an example of what it is that's supposed to be banned—the films never made it into respectable circles in the first place.

Now, that perspective is changing. Not only was this librarian eager for my advice, she was also a bit nervous because her department is competing with heavy-hitter film departments in other universities, each of whom wants to have the finest dirty movie resource library around. They all want the history, the famous court case films, the forgotten auteurs, the legendary performances.

But wait—hold the blue mayo—just as I hung up from our productive conversation, I realized that this library was in fact part of the same university that two years ago rejected a student proposal to have me speak on pornography and American spectatorship. The refusal was thanks to heavy lobbying by "feminist" professors and students who complained about everything from my alleged intellectual poverty to the possibility that campus rape statistics would climb if I were allowed to speak. None of the reasons was put to any kind of scrutiny, because the fact that the subject was pornography made the worth of my contribution laughable: how could something be important that doesn't exist on *any* level of formal campus discussion?

I don't know what happened to the university's "rape statistics," but I'm glad the elitist and prejudiced notions that allowed such a charge to be dreamed up have been sent packing. I'm elated that universities are beginning to include pornography in their sociology and film studies programs. I'd still like to clue them in to the fact that the filmmakers they are so eager to learn about today have not only been unwelcome in academia, but have spent most of their recent years in federal prisons for obscenity convictions—or have disappeared into obscurity and justified paranoia. Even as pornography comes out of the closet, there are still huge class differences in terms of who *talks* about porn and who actually *makes* it.

That gap is now closing. Sexual speech—the place of sex in society—has been injected with a giant dose of reality thanks to AIDS, which has forced people to talk about the big no-no's, sex and

death, whether they care to or not. Americans are more comfortable talking about sex if they have urgent, practical reasons—or a scholarly screen that turns them into social critics, instead of raincoaters with their sex in their hand.

The greatest conversational boon to sexual speech besides AIDS has, ironically, been the feminist antiporn movement. Old-fashioned religious leaders have always railed against sexual expression, but they were from a generation that could only refer to such devilishness euphemistically. Feminists of the 1970s, however, were quite comfortable calling a cunt a cunt, and felt the best way to fight sexism in the media was to reveal it, image by lusty image.

The battle royal between retrofems and sex radicals didn't start because feminists criticized porn as sexist. There isn't an institution alive that doesn't deserve that obvious tag. Would you be shocked if I told you the military was sexist? The banking industry? Your mayor's office? The quarrel among feminists was whether sexist material *that involved fucking and sucking* was a bigger threat to women than the kind of sexist viciousness that happens when everybody keeps his or her clothes on. I don't think so.

Through my critique of Catharine MacKinnon's work ("The Prime of Miss Kitty MacKinnon") and my interviews with Erica Jong ("Better the Devil You Know") and therapist Harriet Lerner ("The Family Jewels"), I hope to reveal the soft fleshy underpinnings of the feminist sex wars.

Racial hatred and fear are right up there with sex when it comes to American political phobias. Few leaders will touch racism directly. Instead of talking about class and race war, we hear breathless monologues about "crime" and midnight basketball. Included in this section are essays I have written about American racial politics and sex: an interview with Elaine Brown, former chair of the Black Panthers ("A Taste of Power"), and one of my very favorite essays, "White Sex," which was written for a *Village Voice* special issue on "White People" (the cover featured a collage of such white celebrities as Roseanne Barr, Elvis Presley, Charlie Manson, Larry Bird, and Wonder Bread).

I loved talking with Elaine Brown because, in true Panther style, she calls everything by its real name. The history of the Black Panthers is subject to the recent revisionism of critics who call them "just another gang." ("Gang" is America's favorite euphemism for black and brown people; it's a way to make the distance between "them" and "us.") I agree with those who believe neighborhood gangs are part of the solution, not the problem. If gang life were not in place, there would be no family, no structure at all. If you think gangs are bad, you haven't seen anarchy. Everybody, at every level, is in some kind of "gang"—it's just that the respectable gangs wear suits and work in skyscrapers and usually don't get their hands on Uzis: they have other effective weapons for protecting their property, accumulating power, or destroying lives. And their mistakes, their "accidents," are just as arbitrary and callous as any street kill.

Mixing race and sex seems to drive both black and white hardliners up the wall. The first time I was ever shaken down by the police, it was because I was partying in mixed company. Two men in blue tied my arms up behind my back and led me through my house, which was full of young people about to sit down for supper. The police said they were looking for a "policeman taken hostage" (*right*—he was in the spaghetti pot), but what they were really looking for was black dick and white pussy, black girls and white boys doing things that make their whole world of superstitious separatism come apart at the seams. One of the cops was looking at me like I'd nailed my mother to the wall—how could I do this to our race?

How could I not? My white skin in America is a racist prison; it's a nightmare of privilege in exchange for total social alienation. Sexual communication is one of the few ways we transgress the gap and make a new faith. It's my honor to try and articulate such a fantastic jump.

Better the Devil You Know: Talking about de Sade, Dworkin, and Miller with Erica Jong

Erica Jong's The Devil at Large *concerns her literary relationship, affection for, and analysis of the prolific and notoriously censored Henry Miller. Miller first contacted Jong when he read her novel* Fear of Flying, *which he thought was marvelous. He wasn't the only one. I remember reading Jong's description of the "zipless fuck" and realizing that this was the dawn of the modern women's erotic novel.*

Miller had something in common with Jong in terms of commanding simultaneous public disdain and admiration. I've had a bit part in that same scenario for the past few years, so I was eager to meet another woman who has made her name as an explicitly erotic and feminist author.

SB: I heard that you were on a panel in New York called "Is Sex Politically Correct?" What did you think of that title? What was the panel all about?

EJ: The panel was my invention. The title was my husband's. I've been incredibly dismayed over the last few years to find feminism increasingly identified with antisexuality, which is really an East Coast phenomenon more than a West Coast phenomenon—

SB: Why do you think that is?

EJ: It has to do with the baleful influence of Andrea Dworkin and Catharine MacKinnon, or their popularization. Andrea's a friend of mine and I have great empathy for her as a person. But feminism is seen by the East Coast media as taking an antisex position. Maybe you're not aware of that here.

SB: Oh, of course we are, but when I travel to the East Coast the force of that opinion is bigger. On the West Coast, it's been a real tug of war, and I even believe that the pro-sex position has carried the day. But in terms of who gets published and who you find represented in the daily papers, it's the Dworkin-MacKinnon position that gets named as "feminist."

EJ: I'm very opposed to that because I feel that they are a tiny minority. Most feminists understand that the First Amendment is our tool. Most feminists would never have joined forces with the Meese commission, as they did. I think that was an incredibly naïve act, a crazy alliance of the evangelical right wing with the forces of Dworkin-MacKinnon. What could they have been thinking? Had they never read the history of censorship? Didn't they know that censorship is always used politically and that it is always used against dissidents? The first dissidents it's used against are sexual dissidents. You look at the Weimar Republic, you look at the rise of National Socialism, you look at censorship going back to Zola and D.H. Lawrence, and it is always about putting down the sexual dissident. So I think Andrea was hopelessly naïve.

SB: She hasn't changed her mind about it; she's not saying, "I was naïve."

EJ: Andrea and I just had a dialogue at the New School, as a matter of fact. It was called "Women on Women." What's interesting about our relationship is that we've agreed to disagree.

SB: That's amazing.

EJ: We have agreed to disagree in the name of sisterhood. We talked about the problem of violence against women in our culture and its relation to pornography, and we still don't agree. But the dialogue was respectful, smart; we dealt with her as a banned writer because she has been a banned writer, we dealt with me as a banned writer, we dealt with women working together, feminists of different stripes finding common ground, which I think is terribly important—

SB: If this is true, your dialogue is precedent-breaking. All the conversations between the radical sex and antiporn factions have been along the lines of the antiporn activists insisting, "You are a bad person, oppressing and demeaning women." And the equivalent reply of the radical sex wing has been to say, "You're a frigid cow." It's become stuck at that, as if we had nothing in common in terms of women's empowerment. Instead, the debate has been so degrading—

EJ: Terribly degrading.

SB: ...that when you tell me you've been able to have any kind of respectful discussion—

EJ: Well, there's a history with Andrea. I got very interested when I read her book *Intercourse*, which basically posits that all intercourse is rape. It's a brilliantly written book. I don't agree that all intercourse is rape, but I'm interested in her as a writer. The *Washington Post* called me up and wanted me to do an article on a writer who I felt had been banned, some subject that had not been written up, and I said, "I want to do a profile of Andrea Dworkin." So I wrote a profile of Andrea saying that I disagreed with her about certain things, but that I was even more appalled at the horrible way that she was trashed. And the *Washington Post* didn't run the piece.

So the article went begging. Eventually Andrea said, "Send it to *Ms.*," and they took it. Since then, because I defended Andrea's right to publish, we became friends. We agreed to disagree about some of the things that we disagree about. I don't believe that pornography causes violence against women. But her points about the way women are treated in society, I agree with totally.

SB: Well, I defend her right to publish. Does that mean we could be friends, too?

EJ: She's a very bright woman.

SB: I know. That's obvious. I've read everything she's published. And I respect that she has the guts to go to the ends of an argument that most people stay liberal about. So much mealy-mouthed complaining about men is annoying. I always say, if you want a complete gender-based analysis of what's wrong with the world, read *Intercourse*.

EJ: I agree with you, and I think that's immensely salutary.

SB: She gets trashed for being like a dyke—

EJ: Fat, wearing overalls—

SB: She gets trashed for being butch, for looking like a bulldagger, and that's why the press is so horrified by what she has to say. Lots of people say horrifying, banal, oppressive, disgusting things, but they fit their gender role more suitably.

EJ: She doesn't conform.

SB: Yeah, exactly.

EJ: She doesn't conform, she has big boobs, she doesn't wear a bra. You know what she's really trashed for, it's the same thing Henry Miller was trashed for: she refuses not to be an anarchist. She maintains her anarchy even in dress. I'm enough of a '60s person to say I think that's fabulous. And the way she's been treated by the press shows me how superficial it is, how women are forced into a very narrow range of physical expression—so narrow, you're not allowed to look over thirty-five. You can walk around and say, "Yes, I'm fifty," as long as you don't look fifty, right?

The problem is, I think, that she's also a danger to the First Amendment. I don't think the ACLU is wrong to censure her for that.

SB: My biggest beef with Dworkin isn't that she assaults freedom of speech, but that she doesn't acknowledge her own fantasies. Why doesn't she come out of the closet as the reincarnation of the Marquis de Sade! When her novel *Ice and Fire* was released I said, "My god, this is the complete retelling of *Justine*, it's the modern day *Justine*. I'm gonna go get *Justine*, I'm gonna compare page for page—"

EJ: Did you write about it?

SB: Yes I did, it was just remarkable to me. If Andrea Dworkin wanted to write pornography, she could just blow everybody else out of the water. If she would take the sexual power that she fights against so much, and move it into her own erotic identity, she'd be unstoppable. My problem with Dworkin is a closet-case problem. So many women like her are overwhelmed by men's sexual aggression, brutality, violence, yet they refuse to acknowledge that women have that same dynamic in themselves—

EJ: You're absolutely right.

SB: ...and that it's in all of us, and some women have it more than others who are more docile, more conventional. Dworkin is certainly not that.

EJ: It's unanalyzed. Totally unanalyzed. I think that's brilliant, and I think that *is* Andrea, but you know she had a pivotal experience during the '60s, during the protest against the Women's House of Detention in New York, when she was put in prison as a protester—

SB: You mean where she was strip-searched, and—

EJ: And raped.

SB: Yes, it's sickening.

EJ: And that has marked her entire identity about abuse of women. It's become her political theme. I wonder if it wouldn't have marked mine or yours as well.

SB: Look, the whole act of rape is the idea of crossing someone else's boundaries and doing what you will with them, with no compassion or feeling about they want. It's like, "I declare war on you, I don't care about you." That's what a rape is, but it also has different individual effects on people, depending on where they're coming from sexually. For a butch woman, which Andrea is, getting violated in that way takes on a meaning that it doesn't have for other kinds of women.

EJ: Why are you saying she's a butch woman? She lives with a man.

SB: I know. That doesn't—

EJ: He's a lovely man, by the way—

SB: I know. I don't care. To me, it's a butch-femme world. A lot of straight women are very butch to me.

EJ: Mmhm.

SB: It doesn't matter who she goes to bed with. But with a butch woman, it's really important not to make her feel like a girl, to make her effeminate. You cannot girly-ize her. When I fuck a butch, I can't insist that she respond like a girl with a capital G, or she will shut down. I can't get inside her no matter how much she wants to be fucked, no matter how much she wants to spread her legs for me.

EJ: Yeah...

SB: I have to respect her butch identity. When a woman like that gets assaulted by a man, there is not only the assault on the body— the lack of consent, and the general brutality of it—it's also that her sexual identity has been humiliated in a very profound kind of way.

EJ: That's fascinating.

SB: Obviously this is only my pop psychology speculation [*laughter*] about Dworkin, but it's the only way I can understand how she—

EJ: I'd love to see a dialogue between you and her. Wouldn't that be fascinating?

SB: She's the only other person I know who, as a tourist, goes to another country and looks for the pornography. When she went to Israel, she talked about looking for Holocaust pornography, that she saw it everywhere she went. I said that's just what *I* would be doing, but of course, we come to different conclusions about the same material.

EJ: What do you think of *Faut-il Brûler Sade? (Must One Burn Sade?)*

SB: I was thinking about it when I was reading your book on Henry Miller, because some hardcore people would accuse you of doing the exact same thing.

EJ: I was very aware of that.

SB: Her book was less defensive than yours because she wasn't faced with the same kind of fundamentalist feminist outcry.

EJ: For feminists to say, "You can't read Henry"—I mean, not even Kate Millett would say that. People popularize Kate by saying, "Let's burn Henry," which I think is an insane response to a book. Kate came to this event at the New School which Andrea and I attended, and she said, "I said years ago that I thought that Henry was a great writer. And everybody picked up on *Sexual Politics* and popularized the wrong thing about it."

The Story of O is another extraordinary book. I reread it once a year. It's such a turn-on to me. And I've tried to analyze why I find it so profoundly erotic. It's really a book about surrender.

SB: Maybe your answer is in that one word.

EJ: Surrender is the secret of everything. The secret of poetry, the secret of life, the secret of sex. You never learn anything unless you surrender yourself to it. People say to me, "*O* is a sexist book," but I don't see it that way. I see it as a book about surrender—sexual surrender and every other kind of surrender.

My new book, *Fear of Fifty*, has a whole chapter of my erotic fantasies, about my sexual fantasies at different stages of my life...I don't care about the critics anymore. I have reached the point, hitting my fiftieth birthday, where everything terrible has been said about me, right? I can't lose. I'm no longer afraid. Can they say something worse than, "She's a mammoth pudenda," which Paul Theroux said in the *New Statesman*?

SB: It's the worst insult, and yet, from the subversive point of view, it's wonderful. I mean, I would love to be called a massive pudenda.

EJ: That's why I quote it—

SB: "I control everything with my massive pudenda—"

EJ: I am the mother goddess.

SB: Yes!

The Family Jewels: Harriet Lerner on Women, Beauty, and Anatomy

Harriet Lerner is the family therapist who brought dancing to psycho-therapy. A clinical psychologist at the Menninger Clinic, she has published two bestsellers, The Dance of Intimacy *and* The Dance of Anger, *which have become classic texts on the psychology of women. Her latest book,* The Dance of Deception, *describes lies, pretense, and truth-telling in women's relationships, from the one-on-one lie of faking orgasm to messages that are unspoken from one generation to the next.*

SB: We've been reading a lot in the news about how American women have lost their minds over their body image: grade-school girls on diets, anorexia and bulimia sweeping college campuses, etc. Now we have feminist critics who have analyzed this situation; like Naomi Wolf—

HL: I haven't read her—

SB: But you know her point of view, which targets the beauty business and fashion magazines that publish unrealistic images of women and thereby create impossible expectations for their readers.

Yet there are other critics who don't fault the beauty business. They point the finger at personal family issues that make young women feel insecure. You know, rejection or criticism from parents and so on.

Do you think the situation is no worse than when you were a teenager, or have we reached some kind of historical apex of obsession with female beauty? Why would any woman torture herself over her looks? Is it just hormones?

HL: It's an interesting question. I have two adolescent boys who are definitely concerned about their looks, but not in that tortured way. The women that I see in therapy, in their thirties and above, are not focused on their looks. That's not what's causing pain in their lives.

SB: It's been just such a focus of feminism lately.

HL: I have worked with teenage girls who are obsessed with food in ways that endanger their health—who get a diagnosis for it. In their case, I would certainly say that it's *not* the fashion magazines. Our culture does overfocus on female appearance. But more importantly, there is intense anxiety in these girls' families, in terms of what's not being talked about, or whatever's not being processed from previous generations. The young woman's feelings about her appearance become a lightning rod that absorbs anxiety from other sources.

It's a very anxious time in society, and adolescent girls, compared to when I was their age, have a more general survival anxiety—about their families, about the planet. Even if they don't articulate it.

SB: How might a young man in a family with a lot of trouble and anxiety absorb that, if food disorders aren't the way he acts it out?

HL: Some feminist once made a quip that when women get anxious they eat and go shopping. And when men get anxious they make a whole war—

SB: Beat somebody up—

HL: ...and really I'd rather have a world in which people eat and go shopping. I think that boys handle anxiety in their families through more emotional distancing—both distancing from their own internal worlds and distancing from the family. They don't handle it as much with the concern about their appearance. Although some aspects of appearance are painful for men, like being very short.

Our culture breeds body shame in women, which is different than concern about appearance. For two decades I've been researching the fact that parents tell boys that they have a penis, which is on the outside, and tell girls they have a vagina, which is on the inside—

SB: Instead of a vulva or a clitoris.

HL: Right, they don't use the word *vulva*. They don't tell them about the clitoris and they don't use the word *labia*. And they misuse the word *vagina* for everything "down there." It's extremely disorienting and mystifying to the girl who discovers this major source of pleasure on the outside for which there's no name. She is given a name for this place which she can't inspect, which is not visible, and which is linked with reproduction, the place where the baby comes out. Boys have something on the outside, with a name, which is not only linked to reproduction, but to pleasure as well.

I've written a lot about this because I think it's linked to larger prohibitions about having an articulated vision of the world, about looking and seeing. I don't think it's a small thing. I interview parents and get these bizarre responses about why they don't tell their daughters what a clitoris is. I see it as a much larger issue that breeds shame and lack of entitlement and confusion—a lack of permission.

This used to get diagnosed as penis envy; it might still get diagnosed as penis envy among some of my colleagues. It's certainly not about being pretty enough.

Being beautiful or pretty gives someone a head start in relationships. It gives someone a good beginning, but that's all it does. Once you have your head start, your good beginning, you're on your own. I look at women who've seen me over the decades in therapy, women who are beautiful and feel beautiful but are not doing better in their marriages or having an easier time with others, male or female. I see a sense of shame, an inability to relax sexually.

SB: The hardest thing for me sexually is to let someone go down on me for as long as they want, without any inhibitions or fussing around or worrying about it, just to part my legs and let it happen.

HL: Not to worry about what they're thinking, or are they wondering, "Why doesn't she come already?" or—

SB: I try to imagine that they're having the time of their lives and I should indulge them. That is an idea that I cultivate because part of me is very tense and uptight about someone being that close to my genitals.

HL: You're unique in terms of your freedom. I have a friend who developed a disease called bistipular adenitis, which has to do with lesions on the labia. I went with her to the clinic, and when the doctor told her about these lesions, she asked to see a picture of them. Of course he was a specialist, and had a picture of the disease. But he did *not* have a picture of the healthy vulva. He had this whole library, and he did not have one photograph of a healthy vulva.

SB: She'd have to get some hardcore pornography.

HL: Right, which didn't even occur to her to do. A couple of women volunteered and said, "Well, you can look at me…but I don't know if I really have a healthy vulva." It struck me that shame comes from that…the secrecy is inextricably linked to shame. I think it makes women absolutely nuts.

A friend of mine who's a therapist in Boston told me a story about a woman who came to see her, a model, very beautiful. She would not allow oral sex. She's heterosexual. When the therapist asked her about that, she said, "There's something wrong with me down there." And the therapist said, "What is that?" And she said. "I have this kind of turkey-wattle stuff." The therapist said, "Well, how do you know that other women don't have this turkey-wattle stuff?" And she just said, "I know 'cause I've seen people at the gym, and everyone else seemed neatly folded up."

This therapist did have some pictures—I think it might have been the Betty Dodson illustrations—and gave them to this patient, who came back elated, saying that she now realized that there were just all kinds of fashions and styles of vulvas. It was one of these unusual situations where she very quickly became comfortable having oral sex with just this little bit of education. And this was an educated woman.

I've been on a campaign for the last two decades to get parents to use correct language with their daughters, and I still have not figured out the extent of the resistance. It is profound.

SB: Well, I've just been teaching my own daughter these words, and I was wondering if she could pronounce *clitoris* because it's a hard word to say, but she does pretty well.

HL: That's interesting because that's one of the reasons that parents will say—

SB: "She can't say that."

HL: I'm told this by the same people who tell their daughters about fallopian tubes.

SB: Let me ask you about secrets, since this was such a big part of the book.

HL: See, I think that's a secret, by the way, I think the clitoris is a family secret.

SB: I remember the first time I ever said some of my own family secrets out loud, and how ludicrous they were. I also remember when I started confiding my family secrets to friends, we found out that all our families had this kind of shameful buried stuff…This isn't abnormal, this is normal. Family secretiveness is not an American phenomena; it isn't only this period in time, it's in all ages. So why do people talk about such families as "dysfunctional," when it seems like it's as natural as breathing to have festering family secrets?

HL: Yes, all families have secrets, dividing those who know from those who don't know. Not all secrets are "bad." Some reflect healthy boundaries and the need for privacy between generations. But there is no family that does not have secrets, and often families are paying for things that happened in previous generations that were never processed or talked about. Every family will have its "high twitch" areas that can't be talked about. You know when it's a hot issue in the family because either people can't talk about it at all or they focus on it incessantly in an anxious, nonproductive manner. The higher the level of chronic anxiety in a family, the more the family will resort to silence and secrecy.

There was this period of time when the recovery movement was big, and women would come over to me and they would say, "Hi, I'm Susie, I'm the adult daughter of a dysfunctional family system." I just couldn't stand it, I can't stand people talking about their "dysfunctional family systems."

First of all, the very term *dysfunctional*, which I once liked, now reminds me of broken stereo components. There's no family that provides for the unfolding of all conversation and for the cultivation of our true, authentic selves and so on. I would agree with you that it is normal for families to have family secrets. However, the fact that something is normal or universal, whether it's secrecy or scapegoating or war—whatever it is that our species does under stress— doesn't mean it's good for us. There's a difference between understanding that something is normal and that we don't have to feel singled out about our dysfunctional family, and thinking that it's good for us.

Parents are able to hide the content of a secret, but they can't hide the emotional intensity surrounding it. And kids have radar. They sense when there's a disturbance in the field, they sense increases of anxiety and tension and distance. When they can't ask what the problem is, they create extraordinary self-blaming fantasies to explain the inexplicable and try to fill in the missing pieces.

A lot of kids will be dragged to me for therapy, where the symptom isn't solved until the facts get out on the table. The term "family secrets" really refers to large content areas like parentage, sexual identity, violence, financial and employment status, etc. Yet you can also have a very trivial secret that has a high cost for a family because it sets up insiders and outsiders and pseudo-bonds between those who know, and who's in which camp and so forth.

SB: A lot of the therapy *du jour* doesn't talk about humankind as a species; it's entirely focused on the individuals and their immediate family relations. But when you compare family troubles to international troubles, where conflict leads to war, that certainly doesn't get treated in a personal way. It's treated politically and philosophically.

HL: Exactly. Nowhere in any of my work is anyone pathologized. Or called "dysfunctional." Or called "sick." Nowhere. There's this huge overfocus on individual pathology and a great deal of parent-blaming for issues that are much larger.

SB: What did you think of the early radical therapy movement in the late '60s? It was more interested in diagnosing capitalism and why it screwed people up than it was in labeling everybody manic-depressive or schizophrenic. Do you remember those—?

HL: Yes, I do. We operate in many different systems. When I learned psychoanalytic theory I thought in terms of the intrapsychic system, everything under our own skin: id, ego, superego.

Then I learned about the family system, and was able to think in terms of family dynamics, and then I learned multigenerational theory, where I was able to see problems in the context of several hundred years.

And then feminism helped me to appreciate that the family doesn't just hang in a vacuum, even a multigenerational family; it's in a context, a society. Any time my perspective is narrowed—when I only see the problem between Mother and little Johnny, but I'm not seeing the generations and the triangles and outside issues—I'm not as effective. When we don't have a larger context, we tend to pathologize. The broader my perspective, the more effective I am in helping people change.

White Sex

"WHITE SEX," I repeated, for the third time. Not "right" sex or "wide" sex or a new drug to do it to, which is what everyone imagined when I announced the subject—everyone being white, of course. So let me spell it out for you: white sex, as in white people and how they fuck, and is there anything to it?

White sex is commonly referred to simply as "sex." Whenever we hear the results of a new survey about how many males over forty-five watch porn videos, or the number of women under thirty who have performed fellatio, we can picture the people behind the statistics clearly enough: white men and women responding to each inquiry, scratching their heads and pressing down hard with their No. 2 pencils.

Perhaps that is our first definition, that white sex is about white people as the erotic yardstick, the arbiters of public taste, the bearers of a terribly self-conscious but largely unspoken standard. White sex at its most transparent is the product of white Protestant or Catholic middle-/working-/no-class, absolutely assimilated, English-First Americans.

Okay, now that we're alone, let's let our hair down, even though as white people that's exactly the thing we find so hard to do. The essence of white sex is sexual blandness and rigidity. Straight white male sexuality in particular is an endless source of folk humor as the bastion of anal retentiveness. An anonymous social critic put it perfectly in the 1960s: "You're nothing but an uptight white asshole."

But why would *anyone* be a tightass, especially a white American male? Perhaps, as we've seen in so many tales about unsatisfied rich (white) Americans, there is something about the work ethic and the American Dream that entails paying an erotic and intimate price for material success. "He who has the most toys wins," reads a popular bumper sticker, but the winner may find he can't get it up anymore.

Or he comes too soon. In either case, the winner, the man in charge, cannot relax. And if you can't relax, you can't get fucked and enjoy it.

What makes white sexuality so dynamic is that, having been strung up as tight as a racket, white lovers are sensitive to the least little provocation. The high watermark of white sex is the white person who loses his or her head and becomes a bona fide sex maniac. As the late cookbook author Ernest Matthew Mickler put it, "I can just hear Raenelle and Betty Sue at every Tupperware party in Rolling Fork saying, 'Ernie went from white trash to WHITE TRASH overnight.' "

Yes, the path from repressed nerd to bohemian libertine is one bright white circle, and it can lead from the first persona to the second as quickly as a whirl of J. Edgar Hoover's slip.

Let's look at a gallery of some of our most stirring White Sex stereotypes:

Yankee Whore: The first time I visited Central America, I had a Spanish instructor who was eager to teach me card games and talk about sex. He told me his last *americana* student had kept a pet boa constrictor that she used as a dildo. He'd heard this was common. He laughed at my protests, knowing I was the voice of reason but delighting more in the titillation of the rumor.

The white woman abroad is the symbol of feminine amorality. She's like that little kid who'll eat anything—except she'll *fuck* anything. She has no shame, she's sexually voracious, and kinky is her middle name.

GWM: Weak, effete, and elite: that's the old-fashioned caricature of well-to-do whiteness as metaphor for male homosexuality. The recipe for being thin, rich, and lily-white seems to have a narcissistic button just waiting to be pushed. It's the "white man gone wrong," which he accomplishes by ditching his family's expectations, though not necessarily his social privilege.

Unlike the straight white male, who can't seem to unclench his jaw or his butt, the out-of-the-closet GWM is pegged as too blatant, too promiscuous, and a blabbermouth besides. The closeted version is just plain scary.

"Fucking white faggot" is one of the most pervasive catcalls of the street, but it is also one of the most outdated. Gay fashion has steadily imitated hyper-butchness, rather than yearning for it, ever since Stonewall. Genderfuck, and consequently gay life, is also getting very unwhite lately, with publicity to boot. The gay diva of the decade is a black snap queen, not a limp (white) wrist.

The Stepford Wife Who Steps Out: If you read your *Winnie the*

Pooh books carefully, you remember that James James Morrison Morrison's notorious mother declared that she was going down to the Edge of the Town for a couple of things—and never returned. In the old days, she probably would have stopped at a dark lounge where a woman in white bucks would offer her a drink. In the modern version, Ms. Morrison is so bored in the suburbs that she enrolls in a women's studies class. In the third week, her teacher addresses the Case of the Married Lesbian. The next thing we know, Jimmy's mom is at the Dinah Shore golf tournament weekend in Palm Springs (does it get any whiter than this?) eating pussy and ecstasy. Her husband and children say they "will never understand what happened."

Once You Go Black, You Never Go Back: There are two classic ways for the white girl to lose her snowy facade: lesbianism and sleeping with black men. I remember in the eleventh grade my friend Carol had been going steady with the same white teenage Marxist-Leninist for six years, and she was in despair. She told me she would be happier with a woman and confided her lesbian intentions, which was a popular pronouncement in Los Angeles circa 1975. But the next night she wound up in South Central with a black Marxist-Leninist man, and she never mentioned the "L-word" again.

To most white people, the most pornographic notion about the attraction of white women (and white homosexuals) to black men is His Enormous Black Cock, the body part she worships like a totem, the one thing that could "fill her up" after years of lackluster intercourse.

But cock-worshipping by itself is no more significant to the "nigger-loving" white girl's wantonness than her lesbian counterpart's purported lust for muff-diving. Miss Anne wants *off* her pedestal because she can't *get* off as long as she's stuck there. She wants to be treated like a Real Woman (say this with an ethnic accent); she wants to submit to "perverts" and "savages," and if it all goes according to cliché, she will earn the degrading, yet elating title of White Bitch in Heat.

When a white woman is called a "nigger-lover," it means that she puts her sexual satisfaction before her racial unity. The crucial thing about this little notion is that white women aren't supposed to put their sexual satisfaction before *anything*. Of course she isn't going back!

Scary White Guys: Ted Bundy. Jeffrey Dahmer. You name it. They seethe, they plot, and they plan. They are said to find inspiration for their sadism from looking at dirty pictures, but more often than not, they say they find their justification in the Bible. Only white men seem to sodomize fourteen children in the neighborhood, mutilate their bodies, and bury them in the back yard. They've got the Psychotic Geek market all wrapped up. In nonwhite families, the cry is heard round the television set: "Our people don't do that." That's not actually true; every race is capable of unspeakable atrocities. White men's sex crimes capture the media eye partly because their white victims get more attention. Look how long Dahmer was ignored by the police because his victims were *not* white. White male serial killers are the ultimate example of repressed white sexuality gone berserk. Prudery, in these men's hands, is a Texas chainsaw.

Let's (Wear Orange and) Get It On: I used to live in an apartment below a Rajneesh commune, its New Age members decked out in tangerine and magenta. Every day and night they practiced floor-pounding primal-scream gymnastics, which they called Chaotic Meditations. (I called the landlord.) Sex inevitably was part of their chaos and often spilled out into our backyard. Outside my bedroom window, I saw a lot of orange in the missionary position.

For commune members, sex was liberated from traditions of getting married and whitebreading it. The men studied massage and vied for Spiritual Leadership, while the women supported the commune through sex work. At one point, I recall, every woman working at one downtown burlesque theater was either a dyke or a Rajneeshi.

"Eastern" eroticism and spiritual quests have been one of the great attempts of white baby boomers to get out from under the White Man's Sexual Burden. To these spiritualists, sexual guilt and shame are disparaged as ridiculous notions of Christianity and Western Civilization. They are, certainly; but the fact that none of the world's religions is exactly an advertisement for sexual liberation was lost on the new cult followers.

Oriental romanticism allows white people to go wild with spiritual pretensions. The right *Kama Sutra* manual could send a devotee over the top of sexual bliss and into enlightenment. Queer and interracial liaisons may be bad for one's reputation, but (at least in California) you can fuck your brains out under the guise of devout prayer and guidance.

White sex is clearly an object of derision both for being hopelessly uptight and completely debauched. The debauchery supposedly comes from outside the white world, but in fact it comes from white lovers yearning to undo themselves. When white people seek their erotic identities, they become fallen angels; but when *non*white people follow some of the same paths, they are criticized by the conservative members of their community for "acting white," i.e., having no moral center. It's an equal opportunity for all colors to bash sexual desire and imagination.

Perhaps the cruelest point of the stereotypes is this: they imply that sexual freedom is a bad end, because one's erotic yearnings can only be quenched at the price of losing one's family ties, morality, and intellectual respectability. Privately, I like to be a White Bitch in Heat, but publicly, it's a total embarrassment. There's the rub, the hypocrisy, the threat to my status as White Lady.

I know I'm not alone in having sex as a Yankee Whore or a Nigger-Lover. White sex will be eroticized by racism and anxieties about sexual deviance as long as inequality remains a cornerstone of our erotic taboos. We can't easily squirm out from under the effects of institutional white power, or the WASP work ethic, or the white picket fence surrounding the nuclear family.

Lust may be blind, but social appearances are painfully discriminating. White sex has not so much suffered from its stereotypes as it has from everyone's pretending that the stereotypes don't exist. A touch of honesty is the only thing that works wonders. Surrender to the debauchery of white sex and watch the fur fly! The truth is, everyone deserves the chance to be a White Bitch in Heat, at least once in a lifetime.

A Taste of Power:
Tasting and Talking with Elaine Brown

*The Panthers were the epitome of Black Power. They were beyond
separatism, and were unabashed revolutionaries. Far to the left of the
antiwar movement, they were Mao-influenced socialists. Panther
Party members carried guns on the city streets in the name of self-* 113
*defense, dogging the white police occupation of the ghetto. No one
would ever call the Panthers social workers, yet they instituted some
of the most meaningful self-help programs inside the black community, dished out in-school breakfast programs, education, and preven-
tive health care projects.*

*In the city of their origin—Oakland, California—the Panthers so
transformed local politics that Lionel Wilson received the votes he
needed to become the city's first black mayor. No one would guess it
today, but mainstream black Democratic Party politics as we know it
would have been unthinkable before the Panthers.*

*As influential as the Panthers were, they were also destroyed inter-
nally by COINTELPRO, a covert operation initiated by J. Edgar Hoover
at the FBI. Panther leaders were set up and assassinated. Their organization was riddled with informers. Party members had their own
honest differences, not to mention raving egos; but the FBI's relentless
disinformation and disruption put one fat nail in their coffin. Started
in 1966 by Huey Newton and Bobby Seale, the Panthers were all but
gone by the mid '70s.*

*As a teenager, I read all the classics by Panther Party members:
Eldridge Cleaver's poetic* Soul On Ice, *George Jackson's stinging letters
from prison, Stokely Carmichael's speeches that could turn a stone into
milk. Huey Newton's famous poster hung on my wall, a photograph of
him seated in a rattan wingback chair, wearing the trademark Panther
black leather jacket and holding a shotgun like an African spear.*

*I myself belonged to a cadre organization in the '70s which was
inspired by the Black Panther Party. Angela Davis, Bobby Seale, and*

Huey Newton were heroes of mine. I wanted to do everything they had done, and outlive the FBI to tell about it.

Like every radical organization of the '60s, the Panthers attracted young women who found themselves in a world that rejected female leadership as thoroughly as any corporate boardroom. But women were told both implicitly and point blank that they were present to serve their men and nurture their children.

I remember finding pictures of Panther women, like Ericka Huggins and Kathleen Cleaver, their arms raised in clenched fists, and staring at them for hours, wondering, "Who are you?" They looked so damn tough.

Elaine Brown was one of those women. She was the first, last, and only woman Chairman of the Panther Party, handpicked by Huey Newton when he fled from a murder rap to exile in Cuba. The day she took over the organization, Brown assembled several hundred Panther cadre in an Oakland auditorium. Her classic opening line is something I love to quote whenever I want to make a strong first impression: "I have all the guns and all the money. I can withstand challenge from without and from within. Am I right, Comrades?"

When Newton returned to the United States, Brown's close relationship with him was threatened by his severe cocaine abuse and by factionalism within the Party. Discipline and retribution had always been harsh inside the Panthers' organization; but with Newton's erratic behavior, the party became a dangerous place for even the most loyal members. Elaine made a critical decision to leave the party and go into hiding.

Brown returned to public life in 1993 with an autobiography entitled A Taste of Power. *After leaving the Panthers, she raised her young daughter to adulthood and moved to northern France.*

As the title of her book suggests, Brown speaks from having had a genuine taste of power. When she says "we" or "us," she invariably means black women, the black community or the Black Panther Party.

I began Elaine's interview by saying that I'd wanted to meet her, the Panther woman with her fist in the sky, for a long, long time....

EB: I've had people say that they didn't know there were women in the Party—'cause they're still at the poster level. There's this whole notion that there were no women in the Party.

SB: Some of the best parts of your book were when you described incidents with other women in the Panthers, like when you toured

North Korea and saw Eldridge Cleaver slapping a pregnant Kathleen Cleaver right in front of you.

EB: Which she's pretty angry about me disclosing.

SB: Why?

EB: It's funny, there are a number of women who haven't dealt with why they accepted so much violence. They're angry that I talked about it. They don't see that they are not to blame.

SB: Whenever you told stories about something that happened to you as a woman that was violent or unfair, a double standard, or whatever—you let the stories say it for themselves. You never wrote, "And then, I discovered sisterhood is beautiful!"

EB: Exactly.

SB: Well, when did that start happening?

EB: Well, we never thought about it at the time. I always say nobody came out of his or her mother's womb with a black consciousness, you know what I mean? But people pretend they have, you know.

I didn't try to pretend that I was somebody else at the time. So when I wrote about being a little girl, I said I wanted to be white. I could have said I wanted to be white because I thought that white was good and black was bad because of poverty—you know, suggested that with all kinds of polemic. But I didn't because I thought I had to take the person reading the book to the same place where I was at the time. When you find these women's issues in my book, it starts from my mother. My mother, of course, was a girl that didn't take no stuff.

I was like every woman in the Party [about feminism]. We really justified our lives by saying, "That's what the white girls say, they got nothing to do with us."

SB: When did that change for you?

EB: I identified a transformation when there was this guy running against me in my first Oakland election. He was saying to people—he had these little coffee klatches—"Look at Elaine Brown, she is a drug user and a murderess and a lesbian."

SB: Well, gee, I don't know what's worse, a lesbian or a murderer.

EB: It really pissed me off. I said, "Well, which is it that you don't like about those three?" So then I started thinking about all the stuff that my mother had done...all of a sudden I heard my mother being really tough, never getting married because men want you to be a certain way, and all of a sudden I heard all these voices of women who have accosted me in the past. I remember one group coming over to the Panther Party office, some radical white women who wanted to use our mimeograph machine, and they said to me, "You are a lackey for men!"

I'm like, "You're in the Black Panther office. It's our mimeograph machine. Listen to this: Out!"

But they were right, you see, even the most radical of them. I had been—not a lackey—but like most women in the world, I had sought power and affirmation and validation and identity through a man. Only when I took over the Party and had no man to back up my decisions, then a man could threaten to isolate me, and he did it by trying to use the social stigma of drugs and lesbianism.

SB: Yes.

EB: I took a couple brothers over and explained to my opponent in the male language that he could understand, "Don't you ever speak my name—you can't even say that you are my opponent. Because we are going to be in your ass." Now this was the language he understood. It's moments like that that I had a taste of power, do you know what I'm saying? Not because I had those brothers, but because I understood what the deal was, and I could deal with it. That's really what it takes to find out what it's about. Not about gender questions only, but about saying: "Now I'm gonna make some decisions." And there's nobody back there that I can turn around and say to: "Is this okay?"

SB: The thing that was startling about your book was that you weren't afraid to talk about what was really going down inside the Party. But at the same time, you maintained your pride about the politics.

EB: That's the part that tears you. On the one hand, you think—

SB: If I hide this, it'll waste the credibility and nobody will believe anything, and if I don't, then I'm a liar!

EB: Exactly. Well, that's why it took me eight years to write this book. Because it was painful. I was just fucking glad to get away [from the Party]. And on the other hand, I hated myself for leaving. I was as much terrified at that moment as I was relieved. And then I was ashamed to be so relieved.

SB: A lot of your story is connected with men that you fell in love with, and who were your mentors in the party. One criticism of you would be, "Well, this woman just slept her way to the top."

EB: I've been asked that—

SB: I'm sure you have—

EB: By men, of course—

SB: I did not jump to that particular conclusion myself because I thought, these men slept with plenty of women in the party, and not all of them ended up Chairman....

EB: You're stealing my answer!

SB: I've been there.

EB: Do you know what a guy said to me at Spelman College? He said, "People have been saying that you slept with Eldridge Cleaver and you slept with Bunchy Carter and you slept with so 'n' so and that's how you arrived at the top."

What did he think "the top" was, a salary increase or something? "At the top" meant I was at the top of the target range, you know? Anyway, he said, "What do you say to that?" And I said, "Well, the first thing I say is, I never slept with Bunchy Carter." [*Laughter.*]

And then I said, "I've slept with more than you've named." The other thing I would say is that Eldridge Cleaver fucked half the women in the Black Panther Party, and Huey slept with the other half. None of those women became Chairman of the party. So I guess that wasn't the criterion—

SB: But you don't discuss what it was about you that gave you leadership qualities.

EB: Well, I could write, so I became the Executive Minister of Information—

SB: But you could have been a great writer and not been able to command attention and respect of the rank and file—

EB: I'm coming from the street, remember.

SB: I know, but a lot of people come from the street.

EB: No, not that can read and write! In other words, Angela [Davis] could write, but she didn't come from the street. I remember her doing everything just like she was in the Party, and they just completely destroyed her. Not only the men, but even some women saying the same thing that some black women did with Anita Hill, you know, "You think you're so cute." And then there was the question of her [light] color, and the question of her coming from academia. She didn't last too long in the Black Panther Party. But you see, I came from the streets, so if somebody said to me, "You bitch," or whatever, I would just do five minutes on their mother, you know. I could get down and dirty, too. Plus, I was doing everything the men were doing. They weren't doing anything I couldn't do.

SB: I always saw two types of women leaders to look up to. There would be the women who were attached to some man and playing a wife's role to him, but they were not political figures by themselves.

EB: No. Living vicariously.

SB: Then there were the younger ones, like me, and we wanted to have sex; I mean, we were sexual young women and we had our desires. I remember how sometimes we'd get blown away so badly by the accusations of "You're a whore," and all that shit. But then we reacted by saying, "Okay, fine, I'm going to be like Joan of Arc. I will sleep with no one. I will work day and night."

EB: I did that for six months.

SB: See, exactly. That's how long it lasted, and then you'd get horny and blow it again.

EB: That's how I got pregnant. I did that. When John and Bunchy were killed [by Ron Karenga's rival black power organization, widely suspected of cooperating with the FBI] I just said, "I do not have the right to have a life, and I have no sexuality, and the only thing I'm going to do is work until I die." It wasn't a joke with me, I really believed that was all I had to do until I met Masai, my daughter's father, and we made love. He convinced me that we might die tomorrow. But I never thought of it as a line, "We might go out tomorrow." Not I, the warrior, 'cause that was another thing. But we might die, so what the hell!

SB: I want to mention some things and have you briefly tell me the first thing that comes to mind, okay?

EB: Go ahead.

SB: Spike Lee.

EB: I'm glad he did *Malcolm X.* I'm not a Spike Lee fan. I'm just glad that he did that film. Even though he did think that it wasn't a film and that it was the real thing—that it was more important than Malcolm. But you have to forgive Spike. He was not the problem. 'Cause life is not a movie. You know what I'm sayin'? It really isn't, and the problem is—I wanna talk about Colin Powell, for example.

SB: Okay, tell me what you think of Colin Powell.

EB: Well, you know, he is probably one of the biggest assholes in the world. [*Laughter.*] But I stay on Colin Powell. I'm glad he's gonna quit, not that I care one way or another. 'Cause they'll just replace him with another clone—but the fact is, what a goddamn insult to black people. Now we know he's also homophobic. In addition to all his other flaws, he's homophobic. He talks about "This is do-able, we're gonna go into Iraq and kick some butt"—and hype about black men, talking about having a monument built to the Buffalo Soldiers, you know about that?

SB: Yes.

EB: And more importantly, being George Bush's friend, already.

SB: What do you think of *The Blackman's Guide to Under-*

standing the Blackwoman?

EB: Oh, you mean that woman who said you had to get beaten up by your man? [*Laughter.*]

That stupid woman Shahrazad, or something? I wish I would see her. I would just give her a taste of her own suggestion. I heard about it, but who would actually spend money to read it in order to get angry about it?

SB: It was a huge seller in the black small press—I mean I got a copy. I had to read aloud from it to my friends, just to hear—

EB: How he slapped that bitch around, and she—

SB: Well, it's a little bit more complicated than that, 'cause it's part of the next thing I was gonna ask you, about New Age cultural nationalism.

EB: New Age nationalism, that's very good. Can I steal that line? Because I'm going to L.A., and I'll probably get asked a lot of questions—

SB: For some people, it's a lifestyle, like what you wear, your diet, or celebrating holidays, like Kwanzaa.

EB: Kwanzaa. What I want to know is this: What are you celebrating? What is this, singing and dancing in slave quarters? What are you talking about? The whole concept of Kwanzaa had to do with a harvest feast, that's all it is. And I don't think that they had a hell of a lot to harvest in Africa. I have nothing to say for those people. Nothing positive, anyway.

SB: Crack.

EB: There are two problems. One is that the people who are using crack and distributing crack cannot stop the flow because the flow doesn't come from them, the flow comes from the CIA-Noriega connection. Whether or not this was intentional towards black people—we have certainly been the greatest users, we are the point of sale. Sad to say. So sale has to stop from the source. My second answer is that the black people who are distributing cocaine in their own communities need to be dealt with, on two levels: one, on the level of simply putting them out of the community, and then offering them some redemption in the form of programs for their lives. Because most of these guys that are doing drugs are saying, "What's the point when you can work at McDonald's or you can sell drugs?" That's not a difficult choice. I wouldn't want McDonald's.

SB: Hip hop.

EB: I've heard rap music all my life in the form of street poems people would say. I don't listen to most of it, it's a whole bunch of antiwoman stuff, you know. I like some of Public Enemy. They dedicated one of their albums to Huey, you know. Most rap artists are owned by Time Warner and other corporations like this. So, I know they will talk that talk, but they're not gonna do anything. Like Ice-T, he says, "I shot the cop," or whatever that is. Then Time Warner tells him not to say it, so he stops saying it. Now imagine. It was embarrassing to me. This is "Time Warner Rap," you know, but it started out as a kind of underground music.

SB: Pretend you are back in Philadelphia right now and you are in a part of town like where you grew up, and you see a fourteen-year-old girl. How do you think she's different from you as a child, or how much is it the same?

EB: What I've said, and what other people have said, is that it's the best of times and it's the worst of times. It's the worst of times because the real conditions are actually worse. We are poorer, relatively. But the consciousness has never been higher. I see girls today—and I can call them girls because I'm old enough—and they'll say, "I won't accept any kind of stuff from a man." I mean they got it so fast it's incredible.

SB: Have you ever had an affair with a woman?

EB: No. I've loved women, though. I love women now. But I had to work through all this stuff, and really think about it very clearly. One of the people that really brought me to that was Huey.

Huey was pretty much a free person. He made everyone read *The Hite Report*. Mao's little red book and *The Hite Report*. We had lessons on this and classes, and he addressed this to the men. Black men are very uptight about sex; I mean there's only certain positions and only so much they're gonna do. And Huey said, "Do you realize that ninety percent of women don't achieve orgasm, and the ones that say they do, half of them are fake?" We would have discussion after discussion, about sexuality between men and women and how it actually plays itself out.

Huey was a very free person. Crazy but free. It just made him hate America even more, because he was so free and it was so restricting, you know. He always said, "Orgasm is pretty easy to achieve 'cause you can do it solo. So I guess that's not the point of sex." And that was a very powerful statement to make among men. Huey really did say, "I'm not a man, I'm not a woman, I'm just a plain boy-child." He really believed that, in the sense that he felt that gender was so outrageous an issue that he couldn't even be a feminist. Oh, I think if he would have been in his right mind in the world today, he would have been a feminist. More than he would have been anything else.

The Prime of Miss Kitty MacKinnon

YES, I HAVE read Catharine MacKinnon's *Only Words*. I'm one of a miserable group of reviewers and legal scholars who forced ourselves to read every word of her rotten prose. Catharine MacKinnon is the preeminent legal scholar and feminist activist battling pornography and defining her issue as the high ground of women's liberation— therefore we all watch her. But even if I adored her politics, I would have to say this book is unreadable. Aside from the fantastic porno- graphic passages ("penises ramming vaginas," etc.), MacKinnon disdains the use of subject-verb in a common sentence. Andrea Dworkin, MacKinnon's collaborator and mutual inspiration, can write up a storm—I ate up *Intercourse* like a box of chocolates. MacKinnon, on the other hand, is the typical academic who must publish but can't write. But it would be unfair to dismiss MacKinnon for her grammar alone. Her content is what rams my vagina and chills me to the bone.

My friend David Ulin says that to review MacKinnon's new book, one simply needs to repeat the title, *Only Words*, as if it were a command. "That sums up her philosophy, don't you think?" he asks me.

It's true that MacKinnon has a deep distrust of anything that isn't literal. She describes the debut of the camera as if it were the creation of the H-bomb: "In the thousands of years of silence, the camera is invented and pictures are made of you while these things [porno- graphic acts] are being done. You hear the camera clicking or whirring as you are being hurt, keeping time to the rhythm of your pain."

Pain and sex have a definitive connection in MacKinnon's view of the world, but you may need her special X-ray specs before you can understand the images around you. She told a reporter at *Lingua Franca*, the *People* magazine of the academic set, "What you need is people who see through literature like Andrea Dworkin, who see through the law, like me, to see through art and create the uncompromised women's visual vocabulary."

Once she dons her incredible powers of observation, no one is let out of the building. The introduction to *Only Words* is written in the second person, as if she were absolutely certain that everyone would identify with her vivid description: "You grow up with your father holding you down and covering your mouth so another man can make a horrible searing pain between your legs. When you are older, your husband ties you to the bed and drips hot wax on your nipples and brings in other men to watch and makes you smile through it. Your doctor will not give you drugs he has addicted you to unless you suck his penis."

Wow! What if none of these things has ever happened to you? What if you start laughing hysterically at the last line because it reminds you of the last time you bummed some Children's Tylenol samples from your toddler's pediatrician, and he never even mentioned your sucking his penis! What if your main violent memories of your childhood are of your mother smacking you in the mouth when she had a bad day at work, and there's no convenient feel-good feminist explanation for it? What if you attended a very interesting workshop about lesbian S/M where you found out exactly what kind of candles you should buy for sex play? (Never buy the colored ones—they really burn.) For that matter, what if you get your legs and bikini line waxed every six weeks?

The presumptions of this second-person tirade are right out of an evangelist's sales manual. Like Muriel Spark's famous character, Miss Jean Brodie—who urged her young students to join Mussolini's cause, while sweeping their hormones into her magnificent wake—MacKinnon's best recruits are virgins and naïfs. Unfortunately, when it comes to pornography, few Americans, especially women, know a damn thing about it, except it's "bad," and MacKinnon can get away with making statements that are right out of *War of the Worlds.*

If, like MacKinnon, you have never been on a porn-movie set, you may actually swallow such whoppers as how, in porn, "actresses are all overwhelmingly...poor, desperate, homeless, pimped women who were sexually abused as children." As prostitute/activist Carol Leigh recently wrote, sex workers "are rejected unless we come around to [MacKinnon's] anti-prostitution philosophy and become 'recovering prostitutes'...We are not misguided women, although Catharine treats us like that."

MacKinnon claims to have the inside scoop on how porn movies are made because of all the anonymous interviews and surveys she's conducted. She reveals, in her usual "are-you-ready-to-be-thoroughly-shocked-and-appalled" tone of voice, that "in pornography, the penis is shown ramming into the woman over and over; this is because it actually was rammed up in the woman over and over...."

I hate to break this to you, Kitty, but that repetitive shot of the penis going in and out of a woman's vagina is usually the same few seconds of film looped over and over, even though the real action on the set was considerably briefer. This is called "editing."

MacKinnon talks about mundane Hollywood filmmaking techniques and makes them sound like a sadistic ritual. She writes, "To look real to the observing camera, the sex acts are to be twisted open, stopped and restarted, positioned and repositioned, the come shot executed by another actor entirely. The women regularly take drugs to get through it." Twist open *what?* Repositioned executions? Stunt penises? Prozac? What the fuck (if you don't mind my using one of MacKinnon's favorite words) is she talking about?

MacKinnon draws a picture of pornographic filmmaking as a montage of concentration-camp documentary, high-fashion fascism, and draconian male conspiracy.

"What pornography does, it does in the real world, not only in the mind," she says. "In pornography, women are gang-raped so they can be filmed...women are hurt and penetrated, tied and gagged, undressed and genitally spread and sprayed with lacquer and water so sex pictures can be made. Only for pornography are women killed to make a sex movie, and it is not the idea of a sex killing that kills them."

Yes, for MacKinnon, porn is snuff and snuff is porn. She acts like it's just business as usual to go down to your corner video store and pick up a copy of an X-rated movie depicting a cinema verité murder. She believes this despite the fact that the origin of her anguish, the original movie titled *Snuff,* was long ago exposed as a fraud, a low-budget horror F/X grossity with a helluva marketing angle.

I remember interviewing the man who came up with the "snuff" ad campaign. Chris Rage was a gay filmmaker who died of AIDS a couple of years ago. "Don't you have any idea what a monster you created?" I asked him. "This wasn't even a porn movie, but it will haunt the X-business for the rest of its days!"

"Well, we didn't know *that,*" he said. "The film was a total mess. We had no idea it would be such a hit—but the sensation was all in the title."

Sometimes I wonder if MacKinnon has simply been driven mad by all the sick things that people do to one another. I, too, recoil in pain and incomprehension whenever I hear about the latest psychopath who has shot his mother, machine-gunned his coworkers, raped his daughter, or slashed a prostitute. I notice that such men are more likely to have read the Bible than pornography, but I do not hold either script responsible for their actions.

If I knew that pictures were responsible, that masturbation and erections are liable for the physical harm caused by these nightmarish men, I would be on MacKinnon's side. Everyone would be on her side—there would be no side at all, and she would be out of a career.

But, in fact, no one honestly understands why men or women become brutal, unfeeling, cold-blooded, or sadistic. It's a far different criticism to note that porn is sexist. So are all commercial media. That's like tasting several glasses of salt water and insisting only one of them is salty. The difference with porn is that it is people fucking, and we live in a world that cannot tolerate that image in public.

MacKinnon has picked up a drum to beat that is already as American as apple pie, the devil-made-me-do-it bandwagon, where every erection is a threat, where sex is men's domain and women's suffering. It's puzzling why she thinks this is radical or iconoclastic. Her work has dovetailed nicely with the work of the most right-wing fanatics in the country. Her influence on legislation as important as the Canadian obscenity statue has resulted in thousands of books and magazines being banned, including authors like myself, Kathy Acker, David Leavitt, and even her dear comrade, Andrea Dworkin. (A Canadian customs official took one look at Dworkin's title, *Woman Hating*, and stupidly using the MacKinnon criterion of banning anything that "degrades women," refused the book entry.)

Yet MacKinnon acts like she is the outcast, the martyr. Her book is published by Harvard University Press—which, as reviewer Jonathan Yardley said in a *Washington Post Book World* review, "is vivid evidence of the very free speech toward which MacKinnon is so cavalier." She has a tenured position at Michigan Law School. She posed for a lovey-dovey pictorial with her paramour Jeffrey Masson on the cover of *New York* magazine in such fawning poses that, even if you didn't know who she and Masson were, you might find your feminist aesthetics turning a little green around the gills. She gets called a genius and a brilliant mind by all sorts of mucky-mucks, and then she has the nerve to act like she's the Harriet Tubman of the underground survivor's network.

Sure, MacKinnon has the ACLU to contend with, and plenty of booksellers are bohemians who are going to argue with her in public. But she has plenty of company among those who are offended by sex, and who believe that what they are offended by should be legislated against. It's the easiest thing in the world to be disgusted by sexuality—we've been raised to do it automatically. It's quite a different matter to embrace sexual diversity or, as a woman, to say that female orgasm is crucial to female power.

MacKinnon has never liberated masturbation. She indicts sexuality like a traditionalist, stating boldly that "Pornography is masturbation material. Men know this."

But what about women? MacKinnon apparently finds the idea that women masturbate, perhaps even using sexy words and pictures, altogether unbelievable—or yet another symptom of a pimp's brainwashing. It's this arrogance and condescension that make women, not men, MacKinnon's fiercest critics and bitterest enemies.

Virtually all men feel slandered by MacKinnon's descriptions of their gender, including a number of the judges she's been up against. But many of them also feel guilty about porn and sex; and when they see the evidence of men who have gone off the deep end, they often privately think to themselves, "There but for the grace of God go I." Such is the nature of the American Puritan mind: men feel that if they could have the pleasure they wanted, they would all go to hell in a hand basket.

Women, by contrast, are so new at creating their own erotic market, so unaccustomed to finding that they can buy a vibrator in any department store in America, that many are eager to come out of the erotic closet. Lusty women have rebelled against the double standard, and they're hardly worried that sex is going to drive them to violence and mayhem.

MacKinnon is utterly disconnected from these women, many of whom are her peers but who are typically of a different generation. The majority of work that MacKinnon's influence has stifled or censored is the work of people under thirty, the "slackers" and generation Xers who publish the 'zines that are thrown out of Canada in the spirit of MacKinnon's beliefs that they degrade women. They are filmmakers who get their work tossed out of galleries because MacKinnon devotees think they are dangerous to women; they are the authors of small press books who are ignored, hidden, or attacked by the doctrinaire school of feminist bookstores.

My friend Roxxie is a perfect example of this feminist generation gap. She talks about MacKinnon as if she were a pair of bell-bottom pants: "Andrea Dworkin and Kitty MacKinnon are just another part of that 1970's trip of finding the perfect theory that explains everything," she says, calling it " 'Everythingism,' the Big Bang theories from the perfect macrobiotic diet to the perfect feminist analysis."

"I don't understand you," I said. "Don't you think people are still looking for answers?"

"What I see is a lot of anger and cynicism...young people feel like all the Boomers' big theories went bust and left a mess. No one buys the crap that there's one self-centered way to look at things anymore. That was a '70s luxury item."

Roxxie is the editor of *Girljock*, a 'zine that is definitely an example of an attitude rather than a solution. *GJ* is inspired by lesbian athletes, but wide open in terms of readership and reactions.

MacKinnon is oceans away from the girljocks, the out-of-the-closet crowd, the rock 'n' roll girls, the bisexual activists, the ACT UP zappers, the twenty-something dadaists who understand *The Brady Bunch* in a way that MacKinnon will never fathom. Because Kitty has nothing positive to say about sexual adventure or imagination, she is cut off from anybody for whom such experience is vital.

Ironically, she is the fiancée of Jeffrey Masson, the author and psychoanalytic critic who has had incredible and numerous sexual adventures of his own. One of his ex-shrinks reportedly described him as "mount[ing] any woman that moved."

Masson considers his sexual past to be like an illness, and he readily applauds MacKinnon's theories—even though he admitted to *New York* reporter Dinitia Smith that he had never read pornography when he was growing up, thereby missing direct contact with the poison MacKinnon describes. He says living with Catharine is like living with God, which I would find rather overwhelming, but which he finds sublime.

MacKinnon herself rarely speaks autobiographically. Tougher cookies than she have eschewed any sort of love life because they could not bear to have that kind of vulnerability exposed. But MacKinnon has been unabashed in her love for Masson, promiscuous past and all. She's proud to be with him, and he fell in love with her, not just because she was a firebrand, but because he could see her as a woman, a sensual woman. "I think Catharine is beautiful," he told Smith. "I don't think that's wrong."

What a curious thing to express in the negative: appreciating your lover's beauty as "not wrong," rather than flat-out *right and natural.*

MacKinnon, too, explains her relationship with Masson with a series of n-words. When Smith asked her how she could justify marriage when she has written that equal relationships between men and women are impossible in an unequal society, MacKinnon answered this way: "Does one not have any relationships simply because society is hierarchical? We do our best. He's not not a man, and I'm not not a woman."

Not not, knock knock. Can MacKinnon extend the same generosity and opportunity to other women to discover how they can be sexually satisfied in a hierarchical society? Can other relationships, a wide variety, be given a chance?

MacKinnon has expressed her conditions for gender relations in a systematic attack on the legal status quo, particularly the First Amendment. It's become a bore to debate the rationale for MacKinnon's legal argument, even though that's exactly what her book is devoted to. She's already been taken to pieces by a cadre of lawyers who think she's a crackpot.

What I'm interested in more is her *cause*. As a lawyer and a political animal, MacKinnon is obviously going to use the tools she knows to win. If I believed that her cause was simply to make the world a safer, egalitarian place for women, I would take her aside and whisper, "I think you've overlooked a few things."

But she's already been asked to listen to other women's ideas of sexual equality and liberation, and she has rejected them. Her declarations are so wild and her righteousness so dense, you can't help but wonder, "What else is at stake here?" When I look at MacKinnon's work, I feel like I'm at the scene of a crime with the physical evidence well in hand, but with an utterly puzzling motive. What is it? Intense ambitions? Opportunism? Bizarre psychosexual underpinnings we'll never discover unless she and Masson marry, break up, and have the divorce trial of the century?

Why is it so important to her not only to stop men from masturbating, but to shut women up? Why do we have to keep our legs crossed for her?

I could criticize pornography until the cows come home, but I will not criticize the power of pictures and words to arouse me: to arouse passion or ideas, erections or damp panties, fears, curiosities, unarticulated yearnings, and odd realizations. Sexual speech, not MacKinnon's speech, is the most repressed and disdained kind of expression in our world, and MacKinnon is no rebel or radical to attack it.

Counselor MacKinnon has not respected sexual speech; she has not found her sexual voice, except to say, quite sincerely, that she is "not not a woman." And perhaps, for Catharine MacKinnon, that is not at all a small thing to admit.

Books from Cleis Press

FICTION

Another Love by Erzsébet Galgóczi.
ISBN: 0-939416-52-2 24.95 cloth;
ISBN: 0-939416-51-4 8.95 paper.

Cosmopolis: Urban Stories by Women edited by Ines Rieder.
ISBN: 0-939416-36-0 24.95 cloth;
ISBN: 0-939416-37-9 9.95 paper.

Dirty Weekend: A Novel of Revenge by Helen Zahavi.
ISBN: 0-939416-85-9 10.95 paper.

A Forbidden Passion by Cristina Peri Rossi.
ISBN: 0-939416-64-0 24.95 cloth;
ISBN: 0-939416-68-9 9.95 paper.

Half a Revolution: Contemporary Fiction by Russian Women edited and translated by Masha Gessen.
ISBN: 1-57344-007-8 $29.95 cloth;
ISBN: 1-57344-006-X $12.95 paper.

In the Garden of Dead Cars by Sybil Claiborne.
ISBN: 0-939416-65-4 24.95 cloth;
ISBN: 0-939416-66-2 9.95 paper.

Night Train To Mother by Ronit Lentin.
ISBN: 0-939416-29-8 24.95 cloth;
ISBN: 0-939416-28-X 9.95 paper.

The One You Call Sister: New Women's Fiction edited by Paula Martinac.
ISBN: 0-939416-30-1 24.95 cloth;
ISBN: 0-939416031-X 9.95 paper.

Only Lawyers Dancing by Jan McKemmish.
ISBN: 0-939416-70-0 24.95 cloth;
ISBN: 0-939416-69-7 9.95 paper.

Unholy Alliances: New Women's Fiction edited by Louise Rafkin.
ISBN: 0-939416-14-X 21.95 cloth;
ISBN: 0-939416-15-8 9.95 paper.

The Wall by Marlen Haushofer.
ISBN: 0-939416-53-0 24.95 cloth;
ISBN: 0-939416-54-9 paper.

We Came All The Way from Cuba So You Could Dress Like This?: Stories by Achy Obejas.
ISBN: 0-939416-92-1 24.95 cloth;
ISBN: 0-939416-93-X 10.95 paper.

LATIN AMERICA

Beyond the Border: A New Age in Latin American Women's Fiction edited by Nora Erro-Peralta and Caridad Silva-Núñez.
ISBN: 0-939416-42-5 24.95 cloth;
ISBN: 0-939416-43-3 12.95 paper.

The Little School: Tales of Disappearance and Survival in Argentina by Alicia Partnoy.
ISBN: 0-939416-08-5 21.95 cloth;
ISBN: 0-939416-07-7 9.95 paper.

Revenge of the Apple by Alicia Partnoy.
ISBN: 0-939416-62-X 24.95 cloth;
ISBN: 0-939416-63-8 8.95 paper.

You Can't Drown the Fire: Latin American Women Writing in Exile edited by Alicia Partnoy.
ISBN: 0-939416-16-6 24.95 cloth;
ISBN: 0-939416-17-4 9.95 paper.

LESBIAN STUDIES

Boomer: Railroad Memoirs by Linda Niemann.
ISBN: 0-939416-55-7 12.95 paper.

The Case of the Good-For-Nothing Girlfriend by Mabel Maney.
ISBN: 0-939416-90-5 24.95 cloth;
ISBN: 0-939416-91-3 10.95 paper.

The Case of the Not-So-Nice Nurse by Mabel Maney.
ISBN: 0-939416-75-1 24.95 cloth;
ISBN: 0-939416-76-X 9.95 paper.

Dagger: On Butch Women edited by Roxxie, Lily Burana, Linnea Due.
ISBN: 0-939416-81-6 29.95 cloth;
ISBN: 0-939416-82-4 14.95 paper.

Daughters of Darkness: Lesbian Vampire Stories edited by Pam Keesey.
ISBN: 0-939416-77-8 24.95 cloth;
ISBN: 0-939416-78-6 9.95 paper.

Different Daughters: A Book by Mothers of Lesbians edited by Louise Rafkin.
ISBN: 0-939416-12-3 21.95 cloth;
ISBN: 0-939416-13-1 9.95 paper.

Different Mothers: Sons & Daughters of Lesbians Talk About Their Lives edited by Louise Rafkin.
ISBN: 0-939416-40-9 24.95 cloth;
ISBN: 0-939416-41-7 9.95 paper.

Dyke Strippers: Lesbian Cartoonists A to Z edited by Roz Warren.
ISBN: 1-57344-009-4 29.95 cloth;
ISBN: 1-57344-008-6 16.95 paper.

Girlfriend Number One: Lesbian Life in the 90s edited by Robin Stevens.
ISBN: 0-939416-79-4 29.95 cloth;
ISBN: 0-939416-8 12.95 paper.

Hothead Paisan: Homicidal Lesbian Terrorist by Diane DiMassa.
ISBN: 0-939416-73-5 14.95 paper.

A Lesbian Love Advisor by Celeste West.
ISBN: 0-939416-27-1 24.95 cloth;
ISBN: 0-939416-26-3 9.95 paper.

Long Way Home: The Odyssey of a Lesbian Mother and Her Children by Jeanne Jullion.
ISBN: 0-939416-05-0 8.95 paper.

More Serious Pleasure: Lesbian Erotic Stories and Poetry edited by the Sheba Collective.
ISBN: 0-939416-48-4 24.95 cloth;
ISBN: 0-939416-47-6 9.95 paper.

The Night Audrey's Vibrator Spoke: A Stonewall Riots Collection by Andrea Natalie.
ISBN: 0-939416-64-6 8.95 paper.

Queer and Pleasant Danger: Writing Out My Life by Louise Rafkin.
ISBN: 0-939416-60-3 24.95 cloth;
ISBN: 0-939416-61-1 9.95 paper.

Rubyfruit Mountain: A Stonewall Riots Collection by Andrea Natalie.
ISBN: 0-939416-74-3 9.95 paper.

Serious Pleasure: Lesbian Erotic Stories and Poetry edited by the Sheba Collective.
ISBN: 0-939416-46-8 24.95 cloth;
ISBN: 0-939416-45-X 9.95 paper.

SEXUAL POLITICS

Good Sex: Real Stories from Real People, second edition, by Julia Hutton.
ISBN: 1-57344-001-9 29.95 cloth;
ISBN: 1-57344-000-0 14.95 paper.

The Good Vibrations Guide to Sex: How to Have Safe, Fun Sex in the '90s by Cathy Winks and Anne Semans.
ISBN: 0-939416-83-2 29.95;
ISBN: 0-939416-84-0 14.95 paper.

Madonnarama: Essays on Sex and Popular Culture edited by Lisa Frank and Paul Smith.
ISBN: 0-939416-72-7 24.95 cloth;
ISBN: 0-939416-71-9 9.95 paper.

Public Sex: The Culture of Radical Sex by Pat Califia.
ISBN: 0-939416-88-3 29.95 cloth;
ISBN: 0-939416-89-1 12.95 paper.

Sex Work: Writings by Women in the Sex Industry edited by Frédérique Delacoste and Priscilla Alexander.
ISBN: 0-939416-10-7 24.95 cloth;
ISBN: 0-939416-11-5 16.95 paper.

Susie Bright's Sexual Reality: A Virtual Sex World Reader by Susie Bright.
ISBN: 0-939416-58-1 24.95 cloth;
ISBN: 0-939416-59-X 9.95 paper.

Susie Bright's Sexwise by Susie Bright.
ISBN: 1-57344-003-5 24.95 cloth;
ISBN: 1-57344-002-7 10.95 paper.

Susie Sexpert's Lesbian Sex World by Susie Bright.
ISBN: 0-939416-34-4 24.95 cloth;
ISBN: 0-939416-35-2 9.95 paper.

REFERENCE

Putting Out: The Essential Publishing Resource Guide For Gay and Lesbian Writers, third edition, by Edisol W. Dotson.
ISBN: 0-939416-86-7 29.95 cloth;
ISBN: 0-939416-87-5 12.95 paper.

POLITICS OF HEALTH

The Absence of the Dead Is Their Way of Appearing by Mary Winfrey Trautmann.
ISBN: 0-939416-04-2 8.95 paper.

AIDS: The Women edited by Ines Rieder and Patricia Ruppelt.
ISBN: 0-939416-20-4 24.95 cloth;
ISBN: 0-939416-21-2 9.95 paper

Don't: A Woman's Word by Elly Danica.
ISBN: 0-939416-23-9 21.95 cloth;
ISBN: 0-939416-22-0 8.95 paper

1 in 3: Women with Cancer Confront an Epidemic edited by Judith Brady.
ISBN: 0-939416-50-6 24.95 cloth;
ISBN: 0-939416-49-2 10.95 paper.

Voices in the Night: Women Speaking About Incest edited by Toni A. H. McNaron and Yarrow Morgan.
ISBN: 0-939416-02-6 9.95 paper.

With the Power of Each Breath: A Disabled Women's Anthology edited by Susan Browne, Debra Connors and Nanci Stern.
ISBN: 0-939416-09-3 24.95 cloth;
ISBN: 0-939416-06-9 10.95 paper.

Woman-Centered Pregnancy and Birth by the Federation of Feminist Women's Health Centers.
ISBN: 0-939416-03-4 11.95 paper.

AUTOBIOGRAPHY, BIOGRAPHY, LETTERS

Peggy Deery: An Irish Family at War by Nell McCafferty.
ISBN: 0-939416-38-7 24.95 cloth;
ISBN: 0-939416-39-5 9.95 paper.

The Shape of Red: Insider/Outsider Reflections by Ruth Hubbard and Margaret Randall.
ISBN: 0-939416-19-0 24.95 cloth;
ISBN: 0-939416-18-2 9.95 paper.

Women & Honor: Some Notes on Lying by Adrienne Rich.
ISBN: 0-939416-44-1 3.95 paper.

ANIMAL RIGHTS

And a Deer's Ear, Eagle's Song and Bear's Grace: Relationships Between Animals and Women edited by Theresa Corrigan and Stephanie T. Hoppe.
ISBN: 0-939416-38-7 24.95 cloth;
ISBN: 0-939416-39-5 9.95 paper.

With a Fly's Eye, Whale's Wit and Woman's Heart: Relationships Between Animals and Women edited by Theresa Corrigan and Stephanie T. Hoppe.
ISBN: 0-939416-24-7 24.95 cloth;
ISBN: 0-939416-25-5 9.95 paper.

ORDERING INFORMATION

Since 1980, Cleis Press has published progressive books by women. We welcome your order and will ship your books as quickly as possible. Individual orders must be prepaid (U.S. dollars only). Please add 15% shipping. Pennsylvania residents add 6% sales tax. Mail orders: Cleis Press, P.O. Box 8933, Pittsburgh PA 15221. MasterCard and Visa orders: include account number, exp. date, and signature. Fax your credit card order to (412) 937-1567. Or, phone us Mon–Fri, 9 am–5 pm EST at (412) 937-1555.